Resistance Band Workout for Seniors

The Only Workout Program with Resistance Bands You'll Ever Need

Free Bonuses from Scott Hamrick

Hi seniors!

My name is Scott Hamrick, and first off, I want to THANK YOU for reading my book.

Now you have a chance to join my exclusive "workout for seniors" email list so you can get the ebook below for free as well as the potential to get more ebooks for seniors for free! Simply click the link below to join.

P.S. Remember that it's 100% free to join the list.

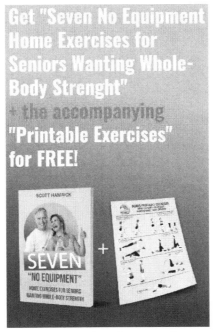

Access your free bonuses here:

https://livetolearn.lpages.co/resistance-band-workout-for-seniors-paperback/

Table of Contents

Introduction

One in every 10 adults over the age of 60 rapidly loses muscle strength with each passing year. The first symptoms of losing strength are the constant feeling of tiredness, aching body pain, and becoming slower when participating in physical activity.

But the thing is that losing strength is completely normal. The average middle-aged person loses up to 3-8% of muscle mass every decade. Muscle loss is also believed to have a big impact on the stability of the joints. Lack of muscle causes stiffness which inevitably leads to joint pain. If left untreated, it can affect the quality of life. Extreme cases can even lead to losing independence.

Of course, being able to run and move heavy things around seems like a superhuman ability after reaching your 60s. But what if you were able to gain that so-called "superhuman" ability back? Well, the good news is... you absolutely can. And the even better news is that you can do it for free... anytime, anywhere. The big secret lies behind the power of the resistance band.

These elastic bands have the same effects as lifting free weights. Combining a resistance band with a couple of exercises rebuilds the muscle mass lost throughout the years. The way this works is pretty simple. When using resistance bands, the muscles in the body go through hypertrophy. This is when the fiber of the muscles gets broken down from the tension applied from the resistance bands.

Technically speaking, the muscles get damaged and ripped. Although this might sound like a bad thing, it's the only way to grow back new muscle and increase strength. Following a 20-minute resistance band workout with good rest and a balanced diet will eventually make these damaged muscles "heal."

The healing process includes new muscle mass developing in these "ripped" areas. The reason why it's so simple to build new muscle is that it takes even the lightest of exercise for hypertrophy to take place.

As surprising as it might seem, rebuilding strength as a senior is not the hard part. The hard part is consistency. Being determined to grab that resistance band is hard. Not because the exercises are too exhausting, or because they are too confusing... NO. Actually, 97% of people admit to feeling their best after a resistance band workout.

The real scientific reason why being consistent is hard is due to the mind precepting this new activity as something strange and unusual. It's not yet part of the daily routine, so both the mind and body try to avoid it at all costs. Now, what happens is that the mind makes 1000 excuses to skip that 20-minute exercise, even though it is conscious of all the long-term benefits. But the thing is, that once you defeat the mind's excuses telling you to skip that workout, you are setting yourself up for effortless success!

The following chapters of this book will not only touch on every aspect of how to build strength and ease muscle pain, but it will also give you a higher ability to persuade your mind on being consistent.

Reminder: The purpose of this book is only to inform and educate readers. It is NOT intended to act as a substitute for curing illnesses or medical diagnoses. DO NOT use this book to get self-diagnosed or self-treated. Always contact your doctor before taking medication, changing your eating habits, or start including a workout in your daily routine.

Chapter 1: The Power of the Resistance Band:

In 1895 a philanthropist named Gustav Gossweiler patented his idea of weird gym equipment for that era. The invention was a stretchy elastic band that would increase muscle resistance during a workout session.

More than a century later, Gossweiler's invention would be used for numerous purposes. Whether it is to ease arthritic pain, gain mobility, reduce the risk of losing balance, or gain back muscle mass. Physical therapists and professional trainers have been recommending resistance bands to their clients for decades. This is because resistance bands have shown to be 2x times more effective than lifting free weights.

For example, when using a 2-pound dumbbell to do a bicep curl, the muscle uses the same amount of resistance from the moment you raise the dumbbell until the curl is finalized. Another thing about free weights is that it doesn't provide continuous muscle tension. As you lower the dumbbell after finishing a biceps curl, it stops further stimulating the muscle. This occurs because the dumbbell is no longer being pulled down by gravity while you drop it to starting position.

On the other hand, holding on to a resistance band with one hand and pulling it with the other will have a completely different impact on the muscle. The more the band is pulled, the more resistance it causes. This happens because, unlike free weights, resistance bands do not solely rely on gravity. In addition, bands put the muscle under constant tension when being used.

With free weights, you can only exercise effectively on a vertical plane. So, say if you were to hold a dumbbell and move it left and right, it would have no effect on the muscle. Relying on gravity is the biggest weak point of free weights as it limits the movement of the body.

Resistance bands give users the freedom of moving their entire body while exercising. A workout using these bands can go as far as allowing your body to twist, sidekick, swing, and bend. Taking different positions while adding resistance to the muscles boosts flexibility and balance while reducing body stiffness and joint pain.

If you're not sure where to start or what type of program would be right for you, this book will help you make a decision. We'll look at some of the benefits of exercising as a senior, as well as some tips on how to stay motivated throughout your fitness journey.

Step 1. Starting your journey

Start slowly and gradually increase your exercise intensity. The more you can do, the better. Start with at least 20 minutes of aerobic or full body workout on 4 to 5 days of the week. This can be done in the comfort of your own home with a resistance band workout routine. If you have not been exercising regularly, start with shorter periods and gradually increase the duration over several weeks until you can exercise at least 30 minutes on most days of the week (or whatever target you set).

Strength training exercises should be done 2 to 3 times a week and should include exercises that work all major muscle groups in your body. Your initial goal should be 10 reps per set. As you get stronger, increase the number of reps until you reach about 15 per set for most exercises (but lower this number if needed).

Step 2 Making the exercise routine, a routine!

In this stage, your goal is to continue with your exercise program at an intensity that is appropriate for your current fitness level. You will still see physical changes because of maintaining a regular exercise routine. The difference is that now you can increase the frequency of your workouts. It is important to remember that even though this stage does not

require as much attention as beginning to workout, it still requires effort on your part.

Step 3 Maintaining

The maintenance stage is an important one because it helps you to maintain the benefits of your exercise program. You have been exercising for 6 months or longer and are continuing to do so as part of your lifestyle.

During this time, you may begin to notice that some of your initial improvements have started to show significantly. These are all natural changes that happen to everyone who exercises regularly. When you're in the maintenance stage, it's important to keep up with your regular exercise schedule as best as possible — so that the problems you once had don't get worse again!

Obstacles

While thinking about your motivations, you will want to consider possible obstacles and plan ways to overcome them. The most common barriers for older adults seem to be:

Lack of time: It's hard to find time for exercise when there is so much else going on in your life. One way around this problem is to schedule regular exercise sessions in your weekly routine. For example, if you know that every Tuesday at 6 pm you're busy with other activities, don't schedule a workout session then! Try scheduling it at 5 pm or 7 pm instead. If necessary, break up your workout into several short sessions throughout the day instead of one long session at the end of the day. Most people find it better to complete a workout first thing in the morning as it not only boosts their energy for the rest of the day, but they also feel less tired than when doing them during the afternoon or evening.

Another reason is that you might think it's too hard or tiring. Well, it's supposed to be! If it wasn't challenging, we wouldn't get any benefit from it. But if you have a goal in mind–such as losing weight–then the exercise will help achieve that goal. The more often you exercise, the easier it gets. You'll notice that it becomes part of your lifestyle and routine after a while. Your body will also adapt so that some activities seem easier than when you first started doing them.

Fear of injury: Many people avoid exercising because they think they might injure themselves if they try something new or do it incorrectly. If you follow proper guidelines when exercising and make sure that everything feels comfortable before proceeding to more difficult movements, your risk of injury should be minimal.

Fear of embarrassment. Maybe you're afraid of being laughed at or ridiculed by others because they might see how out-of-shape (or old) you are compared with other people in their age group of your social circle. Or perhaps they'll just think that everyone else has better bodies than you do — which isn't true anyway! It helps to remember that everyone starts somewhere and has different levels of fitness; there's no need to compare yourself with anyone else!.

Overcoming Obstacles

If you feel stressed out and tired all the time, try this simple technique: Close your eyes and visualize yourself exercising. Imagine yourself running on a beach or doing yoga at the mountains, climbing stairs in a skyscraper, or resistance band training at a comfortable spot in your home. This visualization technique is often used by athletes to prepare for an important competition or event—it helps them mentally prepare for what they have to do physically. You can use it too!

In 1998, the American Journal of Sports Medicine conducted a study about the effectiveness of elastic bands in tennis players. The study showed that out of all the professional tennis players, the ones that consistently used resistance bands in their workout routine had a better ball throwing speed and enhanced shoulder strength compared to players that didn't include bands in their training.

Its high effectiveness and easy-to-use nature make the resistance band the ideal equipment for beginners, people who work out at home, and seniors. They are cost-effective and suitable to fit any lifestyle (even for the most frequent of travelers). Resistance bands come in three shapes:

1. Loop Bands

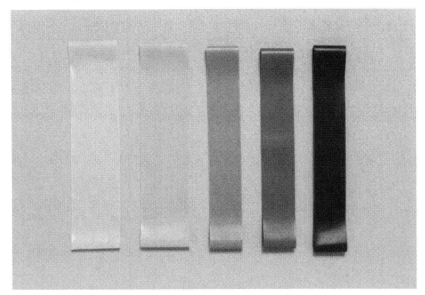

Loop bands have a flat and rubber band-like appearance. They are used mainly for strengthening the lower leg muscles and the upper arms and shoulders.

There are 3 ways to wear the loop band. The most common way is by putting both of your legs inside the band and raising them two inches above your knees. You can also keep the band right above ankle length.

Using a loop band for the lower body works mainly with your glutes. Other secondary muscles that get put to work are the quadriceps, calves, hamstrings, and trunk.

For upper body use, put the loop band around both your arms at wrist length. The colors of the tubes determine the level of resistance the band provides. Usually, the lighter the color of the band the lighter the resistance.

2. Tube bands

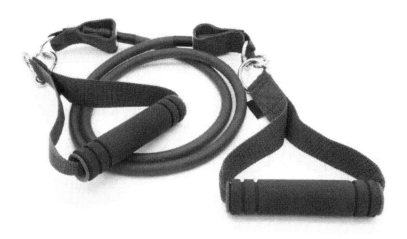

Unlike loop bands, tube bands are set to mimic dumbbells and gym equipment. It is the best solution for people that want the same results without the need of stepping foot outside of the house and the troubles of lifting heavy and complicated machinery at the gym.

Tube bands usually come with two handles; one to hang in place and the other to pull and complete the exercise. You can place the tube band wherever you see fit around the house. Best recommended place that will keep the band intact is at the door handle or a hanger. The level of resistance depends on the thickness of the band. The thicker the tube the higher the resistance.

3. Thera bands

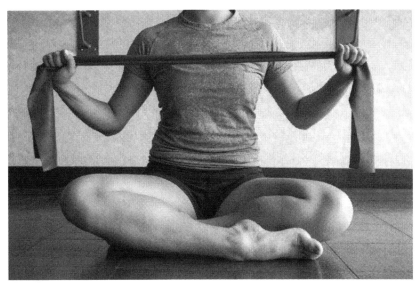

These bands are also known as light therapy bands as they are great if you are trying to gain mobility from an injury or due to age complications. They are highly recommended if you are suffering from body stiffness and joint pain. These bands are light, which makes them perfect for people that want a low-impact workout that delivers results without much resistance.

Thera bands usually range from 6 to 8 feet long. Its length is great for stretching and improving flexibility. The bands work on most muscles in the body by stretching and lightly toning them.

If you are a beginner at using bands, it is recommended to start with a thera band that has a light to medium resistance difficulty. Beginners should be completing an average of 2 hours of light physical activity every week. Two out of seven days should include resistance band workouts with thera bands.

When training with the band as a beginner, the exercise session should last 10-20 minutes. It is important to start slow and awaken the muscles gradually without causing too much trauma. A huge problem with most beginners getting into resistance band exercises is that they get the "rush of the start" where they feel highly motivated and try to double or even triple the amount of activity from the very first few sessions. Some even go as far as using high-difficulty resistance bands right from the start because they believe that will help them reach their goal faster.

But, the truth is far from this belief. Not taking things slowly will just lead to massive muscle aches for the next few days. In most cases when this happens, the body is too sore and tired to do the next day's workout. This increases the chances of being inconsistent and eventually skipping physical activity altogether.

Another reason why starting heavy is not recommended is because it can be fatal. Using a short loop band or a tube band from the very beginning can oftentimes lead to injury. This is because these bands are shorter and put more resistance to the muscle. If the muscles aren't used to it, they can get easily exhausted and let go of the band, causing them to hit the body and injure it. This is comparable to two people pulling a rubber band from opposite ends. When one of them lets go of holding it, the rubber band hits the other person, leaving them in massive pain.

When starting with resistance bands, always be sure to listen to your body. Immediately stop working out if you start feeling dizzy and lightheaded. That stands true when you also feel uneasy, sick, or uncomfortable during the workout. Another time when you should stop exercising is when you feel pain. Although it is normal to feel a slight burn in the muscle area you are stimulating, feeling any other type of pain is not normal.

If any of these three cases happen during a resistance band workout, make sure to talk to a healthcare provider to see if you are physically able to continue using bands in your workout routine.

As your body strengthens in time, you can start to add the difficulty level of the thera band and add a short loop band with the lightest resistance level. Depending on the strength gained after the first few months, you can also try different resistance band shapes and difficulty levels to find which one is the best fit for you. There are three main reasons why you should use resistance bands over the age of 60:

Increased mobility

The biggest problem older adults face is the fact that they start getting stiffer. Getting out of bed in the morning or trying to move after sitting for a long time can feel like a challenge.

These feelings of restriction eventually get eased as the muscles warm up as soon as they start moving. But in most cases, even after the body warms up, the feeling of flexibility is not as close as what it used to be back in the old days. The reason mobility decreases as the body ages are linked to many factors.

The most common reason is age-associated conditions. Some of them include osteoporosis, which is a condition where the bones of the body get significantly reduced in mass and eventually become brittle, osteoarthritis, which happens when the cartilage in the joints gets damaged and osteomalacia which is a condition where the bones get brittle due to the lack of vitamin D in the body.

Although these are three of the most common conditions that impact mobility in adults over 60, the most popular one people face as they age is sarcopenia. The condition causes the bones and muscles of the body to weaken without an external cause. Some symptoms of sarcopenia are loss of mobility, muscle weakness, inflammation of joints, and rheumatoid arthritis.

Unfortunately, studies show that age-related conditions are not the only cause of loss of mobility. Blood also plays a big part. As the body ages, the arteries of the body become stiffer. This stiffness leads to more blood going to the feet. The lack of blood flow in other areas of the body inevitably leads the muscles to weaken.

Another contributing factor to the loss of mobility is the loss of flexibility of ligaments. These are tendons that are naturally relaxed during early adulthood. The main cause of ligaments losing flexibility is the lack of movement of the body over the years.

The good thing is that age-related conditions and complications that cause body stiffness can easily be reduced or even prevented with the use of resistance bands. To maintain or even gain the lost mass over the years, muscles need to be frequently stimulated and put to use. The same is true for the bones. In order to maintain or gain bone density, the bone needs constant stimulation.

When using resistance bands, not only do the muscles and bones get stimulated, but the cartilage of the joints gets put to work more often. When active, the cartilage brings in synovial fluid which makes the movement of the joints easier. Using resistance bands also increases the blood flow throughout the body as it stretches and moves the arteries.

Back in the day, trainers used to motivate their clients to work out by telling them: "Either move it or lose it." That saying also stands true for adults over 60, because you can either decide to stay slightly active and keep your body from disuse or continue losing mobility on higher levels.

Prevent Injury

Falls are the major cause of injury and even death for seniors. In fact, falling and getting injured after is highly common. Based on the Center for Disease Control and Prevention, one in every four senior Americans falls and gets injured every year. This leads to an average of 36 million falls per year.

Unfortunately, out of these 36 million falls, 8 million of them result in serious injuries that require hospitalization. The most frequent injuries include the breaking of the hip, trauma to the head, and a breaking of the arms and legs. Falling and injuries leave tens of thousands of seniors to lose their mobility permanently.

Out of all the age groups, people that are 65 years or older are the most prone to get injured during an accident. Age-related conditions such as all increase the chances of getting injured. Since the bones of the body become more brittle with age, there is a higher chance they can break during a fall. The lack of muscle in the body also increases the chances of accidents occurring. Feeling weak and restricted in body movement will make it more challenging to "think fast" before falling.

When falling, adults in their 20s and 30s have a much better grip to hold on to something to prevent a fall. This is all linked to the fact that they have more muscle mass and joint flexibility. This comparison was made having taken in mind that no matter what, the difference in health between both group ages is significantly different.

But the point stays at the ability to prevent injury. Stimulating and gaining lost muscle mass and bone mass by working out with resistance bands will give your body a better grip to hold on to a nearby object and prevent the fall.

Promote Weight Loss

A lot of people struggle to maintain or lose weight as they get older. And the thing is that many of these people have the same eating habits as they did decades ago, yet they still gain a few extra pounds.

Well, as a person grows older, they burn fewer calories when they are in a sedentary state. This means that doing things like blinking, yawning, and breathing require less energy to continue functioning normally.

Another reason that causes weight gain is that the body's metabolism gets slower. A slower metabolism no longer requires a lot of food. Something that makes gaining weight an even faster process after your 60s is the fact that working out and keeping the body active reduces.

But if this wasn't enough, older adults experience a shift in body composition with each passing year. This shift comes with muscle loss due to an inconsistent or nonexistent workout routine over the years. While the muscle mass reduces, fat mass replaces it. When this occurs, not only do you gain more body fat, but since fat is more metabolically active than muscles are, the body is no longer in need of "that much" food to maintain its weight.

What also causes weight gain with age is the hormonal changes in both men and women. Men lose testosterone levels which causes them to lose drastic muscle mass and therefore store more fat as a replacement. On the other hand, women go through menopause and have changes in many of their hormone levels, which eventually causes weight gain.

Before getting on to the workout, talk to a nutrition specialist or to your local healthcare provider about the amount of caloric intake your body needs to stop gaining weight. The best way to shed these few extra pounds and keep them off is by combining resistance band exercises with cardio exercises. A great routine would be by working out 5 times a week, with 3 times being a 15-20 minute light cardio workout and 2 times being a 20-minute resistance band workout.

Chapter 2: Rehab: Upper Body Pain

Rehab comes in many forms and techniques, but it all leads to the same purpose, which is to maintain or regain day-to-day life abilities. Rehab or better known as rehabilitation improves physical, mental, or even the ability to learn and think more efficiently.

People that seek rehab often have lost one of these abilities due to an injury, disease, or addiction. The reason why it's so popular in today's society is due to it being highly effective for thousands of years.

The earliest proof of rehab treatments was found in ancient China, known as the Cong Fu physical therapy movement. Dating thousands of years back, the Chinese would use rehabilitation to relieve pain caused by injury and disease. Evidence also suggests that the methods would be used by seniors experiencing rapid loss of mobility.

Greeks and Romans also started popularizing rehab around 500 BC - 200 AD. Greek physician Herodicus and Roman physician Galen massively contributed to modernizing and shaping rehab as it is known today. Both physicians believed in the benefits that gymnastic exercises bring to people suffering from physical complications.

These methods were further improved during the 1500s, by philologist-physician Mercurialis. Mercurialis published one of the first medical books ever to be written for rehab called "The Art of Gymnastics" in 1569. He heavily believed that aside from improving physical abilities, people could also prevent them by performing gymnastic exercises consistently.

The 18th century was followed by a boom in science and technology. During this time, Niels Stenson and Joseph Clement Tissot both researched the biometrics of human mobility and came up with a rather surprising discovery for the time. The scientists saw how fast people would heal from a physical injury in two very different conditions.

In one condition, injured patients had to stay on bed rest until recovery, while in the other condition, patients were encouraged to move their bodies through a certain set of physical activities.

The discovery revealed that the patients that performed physical activity after the injury, healed much faster than the ones placed on bed rest. There was also a big difference in mobility between patients who were bed rested and the ones that underwent rehab.

There were clear signs that the injured patients that were on bed rest had lost more mobility while the ones in physical rehab were performing much better, sometimes resulting in better shape than they were before they were injured. This study led Joseph Clement Tissot to publish the book Medical and Surgical Gymnastics in 1780 which would help further popularize rehab even in the western culture.

Rehab is a lengthy process and similar to weight loss, seeing results takes time and dedication. There are three stages the body goes through by using resistance bands as a physical rehab treatment.

The recovery phase.

Unlike the other two stages, recovery is the longest to overcome. This is because it's where the body starts "understanding" that changes are being made to it. Yet again, this is easily comparable to how the body reacts when on a diet. It doesn't start losing body fat right away, but it first starts understanding that changes are being made and starts burning glycogen stored in the liver and muscle before moving forward to excess water weight.

The recovery stage is quite a delicate phase as the body needs to start slowly adapting to the new stretches and exercises. If overdone, muscles or tendons can experience a strain. Strains happen when the muscles and tendons tear or get pulled too much from sudden unexpected activity. Not warming up the body before each physical activity session can also increase the chances of experiencing muscle strains.

Putting too much effort and intensity into the band exercises during the recovery phase might only cause trauma to the body and damage it even more. That is why starting slow is better. During this phase, the body is healing, so it needs a lot of rest. To say the least, the main focus of rehab is not to exercise to tire the body but to stretch it enough for the body to "wake up" and then give it the desired amount of rest to heal.

Resting doesn't always mean lying in bed or on the couch. It also includes applying heat or cold packs to areas that cause pain, reducing stress, keeping peace of mind, avoiding arguments or heated situations, and eating easier-to-digest food.

The repairing phase

After the body has fully adapted to the stretches and physical exercises using the bands, it starts becoming ready to repair itself. This stage is where the body starts gaining some flexibility and becomes less stiff. What happens is that your body tries to recover as much as it can back to how it was before.

The repairing stage is also delicate, which means that the band stretches and exercises should not be overdone. It is advised to stay away from tiring strength training during this time as the body is still in the healing phase. On the other hand, resting as much as before can slowly start being reduced.

Regaining back strength

When the body has restored the painful and stiff areas as much as it could, it is time to include strength exercises in the picture. Increased disuse of the body over the years and the resting phase of rehab both have contributed to the weakening of the muscles.

Now that the body has gotten used to the light resistance band workout you can finally start using heavier bands such as the loop and the tube bands, which add more resistance to the muscles. Also adding new strength exercises to your workout routine will tremendously help in completing this stage successfully.

Rehabilitation is highly important for ages 60 and above as they not only recover physical abilities lost over the years but also prevent further loss of these abilities. Seniors that are most in need of physical rehabilitation are ones suffering from side effects from medical treatments, underwent surgery, or suffer from age progressing conditions and chronic pain.

One of the most frequent problems older adults suffer from is chronic body pain. Body pain is common in almost every individual and varies from person to person. Chronic pain is when an individual suffers from a certain type of body pain for longer than 3 months.

If left untreated, chronic pain can reduce the quality of life and also lead to a loss of mobility in some cases. Three of the most common upper body pain people suffer from are neck, shoulder, and back pain. Keep in mind that when suffering from any type of upper and lower body pain, the body is considered injured.

Injury is only healed through rehabilitation and NOT by strength exercises. Trying to reduce the pain by immediately starting a workout routine might only increase the pain you might be experiencing. Instead, the best thing to do when experiencing pain, stiffness, or weakness in the body is to start slowly with corrective body stretches.

One out of every three seniors has suffered from neck pain at least once. Statistically, women are more prone to develop neck pain than men. This chronic pain only worsens with age. Most people describe neck pain as a constant and irritating feeling around the upper part of the neck or a feeling of tension in the neck muscles.

The biggest cause of neck pain is aging. As the body ages, the spaces in the spine narrow down and lead to increased pain in the neck area. Age also makes the muscles and ligaments of the neck become stiffer and weaker, which increases the chances of injury from moving the head too fast. Weight gain and maintaining a poor posture over the years only aid in worsening the pain.

The good news is that neck pain can be treated with the help of physical therapy using resistance bands. Combining bands with corrective exercises and stretches aims to improve functions of the neck as well as relieve pain. A case study held in Finland discovered that people who used resistance bands to decrease neck pain were four times more successful than the ones doing similar stretching exercises without the use of a band.

Jari Ylinen is a medical doctor who made more in-depth observations on how resistance band exercises eased chronic neck pain. Ylinen took 180 volunteers of different ages, all suffering from chronic neck pain. The volunteers were split into three different groups. The first group would just do simple neck stretching exercises without any added resistance. The second group added resistance bands to the same exercises. The third group, however, was required to avoid any exercises or stretches that included the strengthening of the neck area and were only given a basic workout routine to follow.

The two active groups also added lifting light free weights 2 out of 7 days a week. The exercise using free weights was aimed at working out their chest, shoulders, and arms. After one year, all three groups came back with different results when it came to chronic neck pain improvement.

The group that did no neck strengthening exercises but proceeded to follow a light workout regime had an improved neck movement of 10% and ease of rotation of 10%. Those working out without resistance bands but still doing neck strengthening exercises had a 28% improvement in neck movement and a 29% improvement in neck rotation.

On the other hand, the results of patients that used resistance bands were on a whole other level. Over a year, the group's neck movement had improved by 110% while the ease of rotatability was 80%. Here are some of these exercises you can practice in the comfort of your own home:

Cervical Extension Stretch

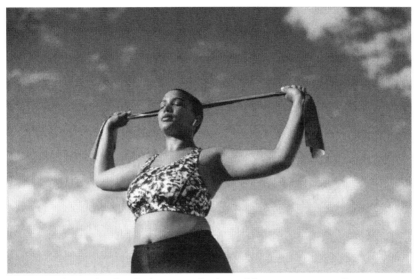

1. Keep the body in a vertical position
2. Place a thera resistance band at the back of your head
3. Grab the ends of the band with your hands and pull them slowly forward
4. During the exercise, keep the elbows in a 90° position and keep your head as straight as possible and your chin tucked and stiff
5. Maintain this position for 10 seconds and then rest
6. Repeat 3-5 times

Cross Cervical Extension Stretch

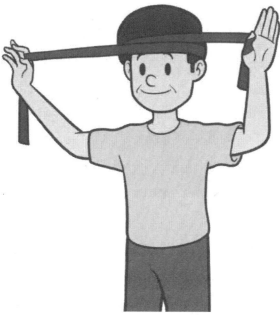

1. While maintaining a vertical position and keeping the thera band at the back of your head, cross the band over your forehead.
2. The only difference this time is that you will grab and pull the left end of the band with your right hand and the right end of the band with your left hand.
3. Keep elbows on the side in a 90° position while keeping your head straight and chin slightly tucked
4. Slowly pull one side of the band slowly outward before proceeding the same way with the other side
5. Maintain this position for 10 seconds and then rest
6. Repeat 3-5 times for each arm

Side Cervical Extension Stretch

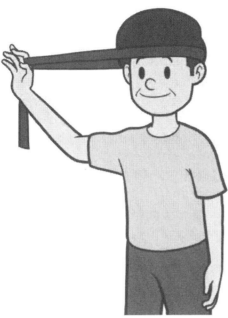

1. Maintain vertical position while wrapping your head with the loop band and grabbing both ends of the band with one hand.
2. Keep the elbow on the side in a 90° position while keeping your head straight and chin slightly tucked
3. Slowly pull the band outward until the elbow reaches a 120° position.
4. Maintain this position for 10 seconds and then rest before practicing the same stretch with the other hand.
5. Repeat 3-5 times for each arm

Keep in mind that not all people are the same. In rare cases, progressing neck pain might be a sign of an underlying condition that needs medical assistance. Make sure to contact your healthcare provider if your neck pain is accompanied by numbness, loss of coordination in the upper arm area, feeling nauseous, dizzy, unwell, extremely stiff, experiencing fever chills, or if the pain keeps getting worse even after taking over the counter medication.

Another common upper body pain is shoulder pain. Unlike any other part of the body, the shoulders are the biggest and most movable joint in our body. They are created by a group of four muscles working together with the help of tendons. The muscles and the tendons as a whole form what is known as the rotator cuff which makes the shoulder one of the most flexible parts of the body.

The most common reason for shoulder pain is due to the tendons getting stuck under the bone area. This occurs from bad posture over the years, or due to disuse of the muscles for a long time. There are many other reasons that cause the rotator cuff to become damaged or inflamed, which eventually leads to pain.

People who suffer from Bursitis, which is a condition that causes the fluid-filled sack of the shoulder to become inflamed. This sack is responsible for the smooth and flexible movement of the joints in the shoulder. So, when experiencing such inflammation, the shoulder area starts experiencing pain.

Lack of physical activity over the years could also cause what is known as the frozen shoulder. This is where the muscles and tendons become weak and lose mobility, causing pain whenever moving the shoulder. There are times when such pain might even come from another upper body part such as the neck.

People that suffer from chronic neck pain often experience some level of shoulder pain. However, this pain is often present only when sitting or lying down and not when moving the muscles.

Unlike neck pain, shoulder pain is a bit more complicated to ease. This is because there are different causes of shoulder pain which require different stretching exercises. Shoulders are more delicate and often require the assistance of a physical therapist to complete the exercise.

Thera bands with light resistance are often the best solution for easing shoulder pain for beginners. They add just the right resistance level to the muscles and prevent the risk of injury. The following are three corrective shoulder stretches you can do at home:

Reverse fly

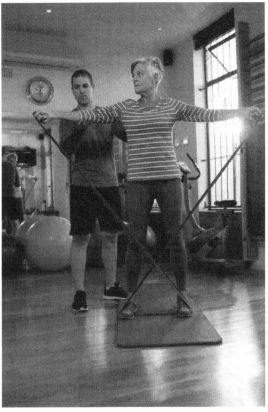

1. Place a thera band on the floor and stand in the middle of the band while keeping your feet shoulder-width apart

2. Cross the ends of the bands by grabbing the right end of it with your left hand and the left end of the band with your right hand

3. Slightly bend your knees and your upper body while making sure that you keep your spine in a relaxed and neutral position.

4. Pull the band outward at chest height with your palms facing down and elbows at 90°

5. Maintain the position for a couple of seconds before slowly returning back to the resting position

6. Repeat the stretch 5-10 times

Lateral raise

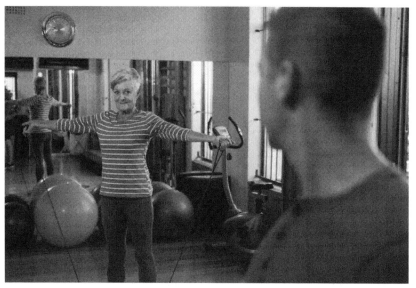

1. Continue standing in the middle of the band with legs open at shoulder-width

2. Straighten your body at a vertical position

3. Grab each end of the loop band with its corresponding hand

4. Keep your arms fully stretched at hip level

5. Pull the band upward by raising your arms to the side at shoulder height

6. Maintain the position for 3 seconds before slowly returning to the resting position

7. Repeat the stretch 5-10 times

Overhead band pull-apart

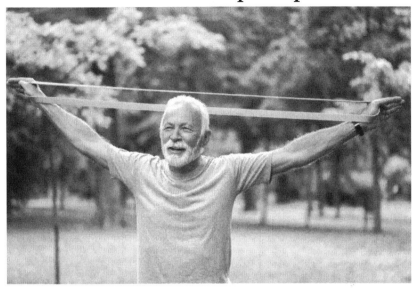

1. Grab your resistance band by both ends and hold it above your head
2. Keep your arms raised in a "Y" position
3. Pull the band outwards while slightly lowering your arms in the process
4. During the stretch keep your head and back straight to keep the shoulder blades down
5. Hold this position for approximately 3 seconds
6. Repeat 5-10 times

Tube bands can also be effective in easing shoulder pain. Sometimes, shoulder pain can be life-threatening. So, knowing when to call a doctor will, in some cases, even save your life. When experiencing sudden shoulder pain on your left side of your body that feels like a crushing sensation or if the pain spreads to your left jaw, arm, neck, or chest, make sure to call 911 and chew on aspirin with little to no water as these are signs of a heart attack.

Other times where you need to seek a healthcare provider is if shoulder pain is accompanied by swelling, redness, or pale bluish color on the shoulder and also if the pain becomes too severe it completely blocks the shoulder from moving.

Chronic arm pain on the other hand is an entirely different story! In fact, arm pain as you age all depends on how much you used them throughout your life. For example, people that have worked in a desk job writing all day will experience a lot more arm complications as they grow older. Unlike most parts of the body, the arms and legs do most of the moving. So, logically, having a good amount of muscle in these areas is crucial for mobility.

If these muscles are rarely put to use, then they will start weakening and shrinking. But, it isn't exactly the lack of muscle that causes pain in the arms. It's due to the injuries that come as a result of weakened muscles that make arms hurt. Arthritis is the most common reason why seniors experience chronic arm pain. The degrading of the joints in the arms leads to swelling and stiffness.

The good news is that healing arm pain does not need as much caution as shoulder pain does. In most cases, the pain goes away by itself in time. However, to heal the injuries that cause such pain you can always practice these corrective arm stretches.

Bow and Arrow

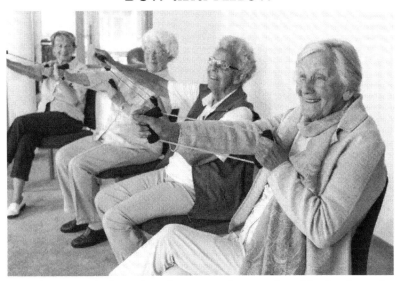

1. Sit on a chair and grab your resistance band by both ends
2. Hold one arm straight in front of your face at a 120° and the other one in front of your chest like you are about to pull an arrow
3. Imagine if the loop band is a bow and pull on it while keeping the straight arm in a stiff position
4. Maintain the position for 5-10 seconds
5. Repeat the stretch 3-5 times for each arm

Bicep Curl

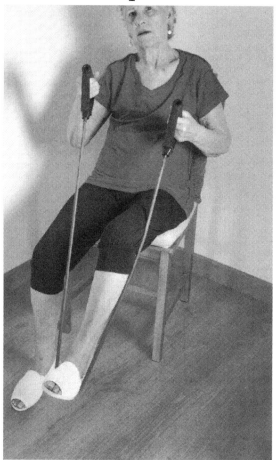

1. As you sit on a chair, place the tube or thera band on the floor and step in the middle of it

2. Grab each end of the loop band with its corresponding hand

3. Pull the band while keeping your palms facing up and your elbows at a 90° angle

4. Take turns pulling the band with each hand separately

5. Gently go to starting position as soon as you finish a full bicep curl

6. Repeat the stretch 8 times for each arm

Overhead triceps extension

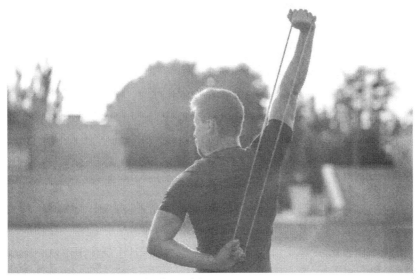

1. Stand in a vertical position
2. Wrap one end of your loop band with one hand while keeping your elbow at a 90° angle and place the hand behind your head
3. Put your other hand behind your back and grab the other end of the band
4. Pull the band with the arm placed behind your back until the arm is almost straight (Reminder: DO NOT straighten the arm fully as it increases the chances of injury)
5. Gently go to starting position as soon as you finish a full stretch
6. Repeat the stretch 5 times for each arm

And last but not least is back pain, which is the most common chronic pain among humans. According to statistics, back pain is one of the main reasons people end up seeing a doctor, miss important events, or even skip work. Chronic back pain can happen to adults of all ages, but unfortunately, it worsens with age. As the body gets older, the spinal structure and joints located in the back get damaged. This causes burning and exhausting pain throughout the entirety of the lumbar area of the spine.

One of the most common age-related conditions that cause back pain is degenerative arthritis, also known as arthritis of the spine. As the body ages, the cartilage that is present in the facet joint of the spine gets broken down. The breakdown of this cartilage starts as early as 15 years of age and never stops.

However, the amount that is broken down differs from person to person, as studies show that healthier people who work out regularly have a much slower breakdown process. Genetics also plays a significant role in developing degenerative arthritis.

86% of adults over the age of 60 suffer from this condition. Arthritis of the spine usually causes the most back pain during the morning and night, which can cause trouble sleeping. People suffering from the condition also experience intermittent aching of the back throughout the day or experience loss of mobility and stiffness of the back.

If left untreated, back pain can become fatal and affect the sciatic nerve located on the leg. Depending on how much the nerve is irritated, the symptoms can be as extreme as feeling massive pain when moving or walking. In some individuals, the pain becomes so severe it leads to temporary loss of mobility.

Because back pain is extremely common, it is not preventable. However, stopping the pain from progressing and also easing pain to some extent is possible with the proper rehabilitation exercises. Adding resistance to the back muscles increases strength in the lower back area. The stretches mentioned down below increase flexibility, ease the pain, and overall improve the quality of life.

Single Arm Stretch

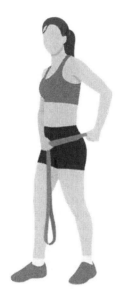 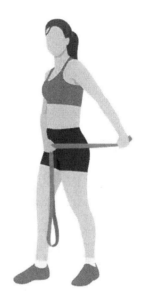

1. Stand in a vertical position and place one leg slightly forward

2. Take a short thera band or tube band and place grab it at both ends

3. Put your right hand on your left thigh or your left hand on your right thigh

4. Pull your left hand sideways while maintaining the elbow at a 90° angle

5. Hold the position for 2 seconds and bring the arm back to the resting position

6. Repeat 8 times for each arm

Seated Row

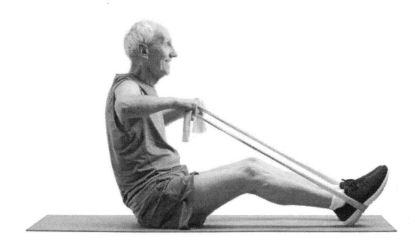

1. Sit on the ground (preferably on a yoga matt) and place a loop band around the feet
2. Make sure to wear athletic shoes and use a flat loop band with a low resistance to prevent injury
3. Grab each end of the band with the corresponding hand
4. Keep elbow at 90° angle at all times during the stretch
5. Pull the band until your hands reach your core/chest area
6. Hold the position for 2 seconds before slowly going back to starting position
7. Repeat the stretch 10 times

Cat/Cow Stretch

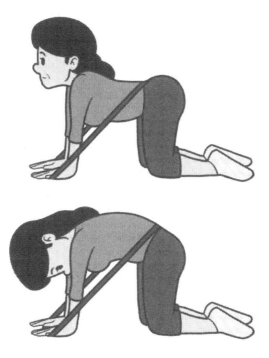

1. Place a long loop resistance band over your lower back and wrap each end of the band with the corresponding hand
2. Put both hands and knees on the ground while keeping your back relaxed
3. Inhale deeply before starting the stretch
4. Round your spine and tighten your belly in an upward curl position as you exhale
5. Then proceed to inhale and arch your spine while letting your belly loose
6. Repeat this stretch 8 times

It is important to keep in mind to call a medical professional if back pain gets worse even after taking over-the-counter medication. You should also call a doctor if you experience back pain along with unexplained weight loss, fever, or problems with bowel movements and urination.

Chapter 3: Rehab: Lower Body Pain:

Statistics show that by 2030, more than 25% of the U.S population will be aged 65 or older. Europe will also be experiencing similar growing numbers of seniors over the next decade. Although there are many causes why there is an increase in the elderly population, two of the most dominant ones are the decline in birth rates and most importantly the fact that life expectancy has increased.

The cause of higher life expectancy isn't because of healthcare and medicine evolving more than how both generation z and boomers managed their health. A study conducted by Blue Cross Blue Shield came to an interesting conclusion where researchers discovered that the younger generation had a much higher mortality rate than the older generation. This comes from a series of different factors.

One of the main reasons why generation z and boomers will live healthier and longer lives are due to their lifestyle. Having had a better work-life balance, active social life, and being less exposed to tempting processed food led these two generations to have lower rates of psychotic conditions, type 2 diabetes, severe depression, and endocrine conditions.

According to statistics, adults 60 and older are highly interested in gaining as much knowledge in maintaining their health further. They are more prone to watching what type of food they consume, learn about how their body and its functions, and are more concerned about their physical health. But despite living in better health conditions than the newer generations, chronic pain is inevitable among the older adult population.

More than half of the entire population over 60 years of age have experienced some sort of chronic pain, stiffness, and muscle weakness. This number only gets worse with 80% of the population over 70 years old having taken some sort of pain-killing medication throughout their senior years.

Chronic body pain generates over 100 billion dollars a year as it is one of the worst public health issues seniors face. Data indicated that almost half of patients who were experiencing body pain had worsened symptoms 6 months later. The cause of all this pain is linked to a condition that affects one in four older adults called chronic musculoskeletal pain or CMP.

CMP affects both the upper and lower body but affects the hip and knee area more severely. A study on the elderly living in retirement homes found that 90% of them had suffered from chronic lower body pain throughout their senior years. However, out of this 90%, 41% of them claimed to have experienced worsened symptoms that even led to unbearable pain and loss of mobility. It was later found that the majority of the older adults suffering unbearable pain were due to having CPM. The main cause of CPM progression is strongly linked to the disuse of the body.

Unfortunately, this condition has no cure, but seniors that started physical therapy and then continued to exercise had massive results when it came to pain relief and gaining more mobility. Starting off with light stretches using thera resistance bands and progressing by adding more workouts is proven to be the most effective way to prevent CMP from taking charge of your body. Three of the most chronic lower body pain people suffer from are hip, knees, and feet.

Hips are known for being more durable when it comes to pain and stiffness. This is mostly caused by the way it is built. The hip has the body's largest joint, and since it's bigger, it allows for more fluid movement.

But aging is far more powerful than any part of our body, no matter how durable it is. With that being said, even hips get damaged with age. Aging leads the cartilage existing in the joints of the hips to become more damaged. The muscles eventually lose their strength and bones become fragile. One thing leads to another up until the point where hips can become a threat to life.

A shocking number of senior deaths occur because of the hips. In fact, one-third of seniors that suffer a hip fracture pass away within 12 months of the injury. Older adults that have weak hips are five times more likely to die because of hip fractures than ones that have healthier hips. Although being a more durable part of the body, once damaged, hips will significantly reduce the quality of life, causing ongoing and unbearable pain accompanied by loss of mobility.

Osteoporosis is the lead factor that causes weakness of the hip and increases the chances of fracture. But as mentioned in chapter one, osteoporosis is manageable by stimulating and gaining bone mass by following a resistance band stretching workout routine. Apart from hip fractures, older people also develop sore hips which are caused by a couple of different age-related conditions.

People suffering from rheumatoid arthritis have the highest chances of hip pain. Rheumatoid arthritis causes inflammation of the hip joint and eventually leads to worsening pain if left untreated. The condition is oftentimes followed by loss of range of motion and stiffness of the hips. There are also cases where people have developed a limp from ongoing and untreated hip pain.

Unsuspected movement of the hip can also cause muscle strains or tendon strains. This leads them to become inflamed and prevents the hip from moving as it used to. The good news is that hip complications caused by muscle or tendon strains can easily be fixable by following simple stretches that heal and tighten hip muscles.

Hip pain is often associated with a set of different symptoms such as discomfort in areas of the joint, thigh, buttocks, and groin. If you want to prevent hip pain altogether before it occurs then staying active will reduce the risk of experiencing such complications as you age. However, if you are experiencing hip pain, a careful rehabilitation process is a must to overcome it.

One thing that is important to keep in mind is that exercising while experiencing hip pain is dangerous and even life-threatening. The only way to recover your hip is by corrective stretching of the hip with the help of loop resistance bands. Some stretching exercises you can practice are:

Clam Shells

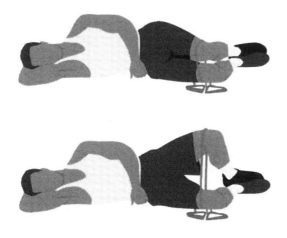

1. Place your legs inside a short loop band and lift the band slightly above the knee
2. Lie on your side with knees and hips slightly bent
3. Slowly open your thighs while keeping your heels together
4. Gently go to starting position as soon as you finish the stretch
5. When switching sides, AVOID using your back. Instead, use your upper body weight to reduce the risk of injury
6. Repeat the stretch 10-15 times on each side

Hip Abduction

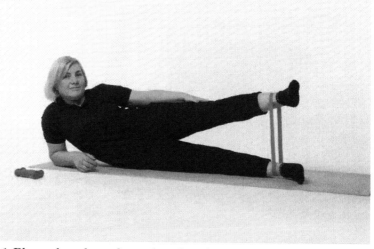

1. Place the short loop band a few inches under the knee while continuing to lie on the side

2. Straighten your legs and hips while placing your elbow on the ground to support your upper body

3. Pull the band upward with the leg that isn't touching the ground

4. Slowly come down to resting position

5. Repeat 8 times on each leg

Hip Bridges

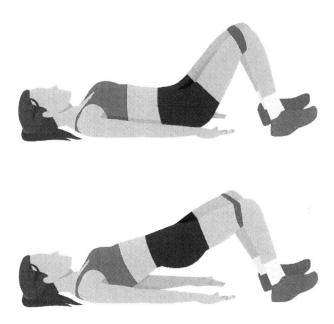

1.Place the short loop band around the knees

2.Lie in a flat in a relaxed position on the ground

3.Bend your knees halfway and keep them at shoulder-width

4.Then slowly lift your rear and gently come down again

5.Repeat the stretch 15 times

While performing regular daily stretches to heal hip pain, additional methods to ease the pain is by applying an ice pack to the hip area for a couple of minutes. Repeat this a couple of times a day to reduce inflammation until you start feeling better. If you are not a fan of cold icy packs touching your body then you can heat the painful area for a couple of minutes several times a day.

Another tip that helps a lot in the healing process is taking a warm shower before starting the corrective stretches. This will warm up the muscles and open up the arteries for better blood flow which will lessen the pain while stretching.

If the pain gets worse while performing stretches, feel a sudden blocking sensation around your hips, or experience sudden sharp pain, stop immediately and seek help from a healthcare provider. There are a handful of cases where people that have developed hip pain were unaware that their hip was fractured. In fact, it's best recommended to see a doctor as soon as hip pain occurs and get advice from a medical professional on the best road to recovery.

Knee pain is another common chronic pain that affects older adults. The pain can develop in different forms, with the most common ones being due to sudden injury or damaged cartilage of the joints. Your weight can also play a tremendous role in the development of knee pain. People who are overweight have a far greater risk of developing this kind of pain.

Being overweight exhausts the joints of the knees. The added pressure of the extra weight eventually starts damaging the knee joints up to the point where every step you take will become more challenging.

The truth is that your joints can hold up to four times your body weight until they collapse. So, for example, if your ideal weight is around 150 pounds (11.7 stone), your knees can hold up to 600 pounds (42.8 stone) before collapsing. That is why most morbidly obese people weighing 400 pounds or more start losing their mobility when they start reaching that weight. With every 10 pounds gained, the pressure that the knee joints hold is an additional 40 pounds more.

The bright side is that knee pain can be taken care of by following just a few simple tips and stretches. If you are in the starting phases of developing knee pain, lower the amount of exercise and focus more on stretching workouts with a loop resistance band. Try wearing running shoes that have good cushioning and that fit comfortably during your stretches as they will better support the knees and prevent them from experiencing too much-added pressure.

Seated Knee Extension

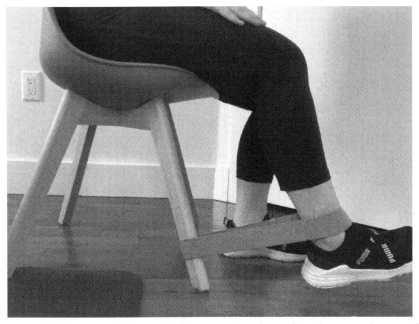

1. Sit on a chair and place a short loop band around one of the front legs of the chair
2. Put one leg inside the loop band at ankle level
3. Pull the band with your leg until it's slightly straightened
4. Hold the position for 3 seconds
5. Repeat 3-5 times for each leg

Crab Walk with Resistance Band

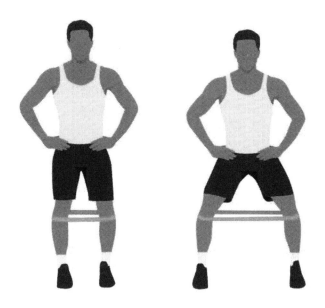

1. Place your legs inside a loop band and lift the band slightly above the knee

2. Hold a vertical posture with slightly bent knees and back while keeping your hands on your hips

3. Gently move one step sideways to open the legs even wider

4. Follow along with the other leg to narrow down the gap between the legs (Reminder: DO NOT close the legs fully for this stretch)

5. Do the stretch 8 times for each leg

Standing Leg Side Raises

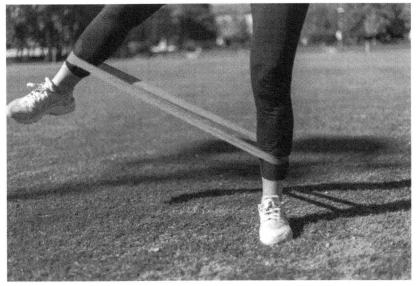

1. Place a short loop band around your ankles
2. Make sure to hold on to something, like a chair for balance
3. Keep your hips and shoulders facing slightly forward
4. Slowly pull the band sideways with your ankle while keeping your other leg slightly bent
5. Hold the position for 3 seconds before gently coming back to the resting position
6. Repeat 5 times for each leg

You can also ease knee pain by applying ice or heat in the painful area a few times a day. Never treat knee pain by yourself if the pain is caused by a recent injury. Also, it is best to call a medical professional if the knee pain on your knee continues even after you treat it at home for three days. If you have pain even when the knee is resting, your knee is deformed, makes a clicking noise when walking, becomes a red color, or doesn't open all the way out then it's best to see a doctor.

On the other hand, chronic ankle pain is caused by completely different factors. In most cases, you can predict if you are going to suffer from weak ankles as you age. This is because ankle pain is caused by how many times the ankle has been injured throughout your whole life. A percentage of the population sprain or injure their ankle a few times during their life. This causes the muscles and ligaments of the ankles to get damaged. In some cases, if the ankle doesn't get proper treatment after an injury, it can get permanently damaged.

Of course, the damage is not enough to leave an adult disabled, however, it does come to haunt you as you get older with chronic ankle instability or CAI. The condition affects 20% of people that have severely sprained or injured their ankle at some point in their lives. CAI causes the ankle to randomly roll to the side or become wobbly which increases the chances of an ankle injury and falls. CAI can be treatable by taking prescribed medication and corrective ankle stretches.

Another reason that causes ankle pain might be the fact that you are not wearing the right type of footwear. Wearing shoes that are too narrow, heavy, flat, or tight can cause many complications for the ankle. Investing in at least two pairs of shoes with supportive foam and a shock-absorbing midsole will make a huge difference.

Around 33% of adults 65 or older develop diabetes. Almost half of them suffer from diabetic peripheral neuropathy, which is a nerve complication that causes ongoing pain in the ankles. The condition also makes you lose some sense of coordination which increases the chances of falling and spraining the ankle.

The good news is that consistent ankle stretches with resistance bands will strengthen the muscles and bones of the ankles. The stretches will reduce pain and lower the chances of injury caused by weak ankles. The following includes three ways to heal damaged ankles.

Ankle Plantarflexion

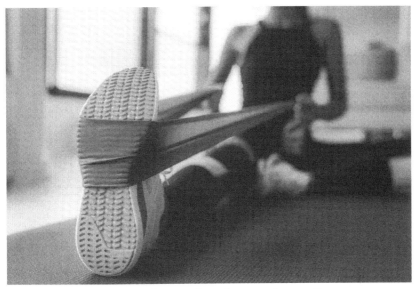

1.Place a loop resistance band around your foot.
2.Grab the ends of the band with both hands.
3.Pull the band towards the body and let your ankle slowly raise and your hamstrings. stretch.
4.Repeat 8 times on each ankle.

Inward Ankle Rotation

1.Starting position	2. Inward rotated foot

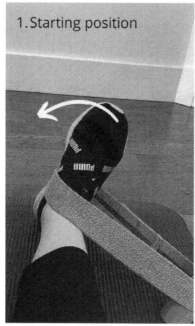 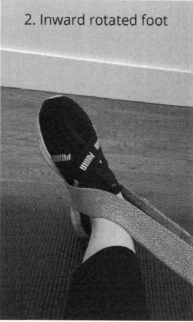

1. Tie one end of a loop band to the leg of a table or bed.

2. Sit on a yoga mat and open your legs.

3. Move your foot inward in a circular motion while keeping the heel touching the ground at all times (Reminder: the stretch will NOT be effective if you pull the entire foot inward. Focus on moving the ankle rather than any other part of the foot).

4. Gently go to the starting position as soon as you finish a full stretch.

5. Repeat the stretch 8 times for each ankle.

Outward Ankle Rotation

1. Starting position	2. Outward rotated foot

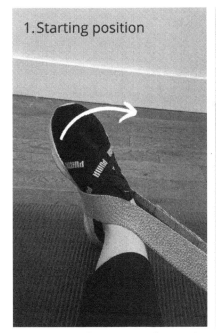 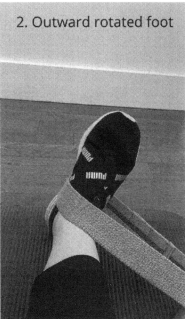

1. For the outward rotation keep the same position as the inward rotation stretch.

2. Move your foot outward without moving the heel.

3. Also, repeat this stretch 8 times for each ankle.

If the pain doesn't get better within the first three days of practicing the stretches or if your ankle hurts even more while doing the movement with the band, it is best to talk to go see your doctor. You should also call a doctor if your ankle gets swollen for more than a few days, and turns bluish, red, or purple. Such signs indicate that your ankle might have experienced some kind of injury, or are symptoms of diabetes.

NOTE: DO NOT practice any of the mentioned ankle exercises if you have recently sprained your ankle and it has swollen. Instead, apply only ice (no heat) on the swollen area and get the ankle checked at a medical center.

And last but not least, is the most complex part of the body; the foot. It is made up of 26 bones and 33 joints working together with the help of over 120 pieces of individual muscles, tendons, and nerves. The foot's complexity allows it to bear your whole body weight, keep balance while walking, and is responsible for shock absorption.

But as you age, the feet get "worn out" and eventually become prone to numerous problems. In time, the sole also starts wearing down. It becomes wider and flatter, which causes pain when walking. Foot pain is caused by living a sedentary lifestyle, using unsupportive shoes, wearing heels, or obesity. Follow these essential foot stretches to prevent further foot problems and ease the pain:

Foot Pull-Ups

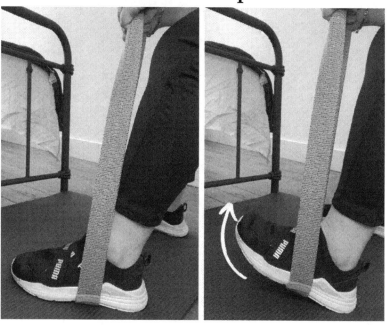

1. Secure a loop band under one foot by wrapping it around two or three times.

2. Make sure the loop band stays in the middle of the heel and toes of the foot.

3. Grab the band with both hands tight and firm.

4. Keep the heel of the foot you are stretching on the floor while slowly raising the front part. up.

5. Repeat the stretch 15 times with two sets on the foot that causes pain.

Foot Push Downs

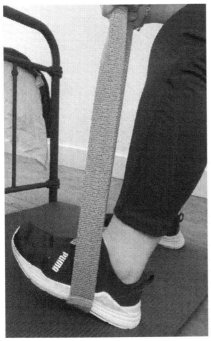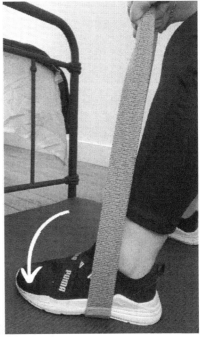

1. This stretch is almost identical to the foot push-ups. The only difference lies in the movement of the foot.

2. For the push downs, instead of raising the foot, you are going to aim at lowering the foot down.

3. This means that the starting position of this stretch will be keeping your heel on the floor and your foot upwards while slowly lowering it.

4. Repeat the stretch 15 times with two sets on the foot that causes pain.

Foot Turn Outs

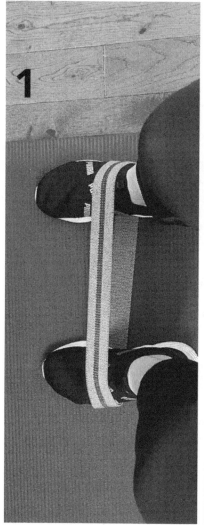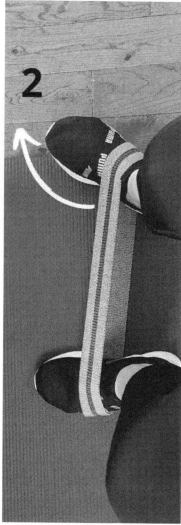

1.Continue keeping the band wrapped on the targeted foot and the remainder of the band hooked by your other foot

2.Pull the band to the side using the foot you are targeting

3.Make sure that the heel doesn't move and remains in contact with the ground at all times throughout the stretch

4.Repeat the stretch 15 times with two sets

Chapter 4: Resistance Bands and Yoga

You might be thinking, "I can't do yoga, I can't even reach my knees, let alone my toes!" Well, as shocking as this might seem, practicing yoga as an older adult doesn't have to turn you into one of those freaky circus acrobats. Many people are left with the impression that the main purpose of yoga is to make the body reach new limits in terms of flexibility. But the truth is, that's not the case. The lack of flexibility you have in yoga is your greatest advantage!

The truth is that being too flexible or hypermobile can be a bad thing when practicing yoga. Hypermobility is more frequent in young adults and rare in adults over 60. But according to plenty of yoga instructors, being able to naturally reach your feet and do a full leg split effortlessly leads to looseness of the joints that causes hypermobile people to develop pain and even cause injury as they get older.

Yoga is not about reaching new records of flexibility. It's more about breathing techniques, muscle strengthening, and corrective stretches for improved motion, stability, and prevention of chronic pain. People who practice yoga with resistance bands have revealed that they experience a feeling of "being held together" and increase muscle strength.

The reason yoga is more beneficial using resistance bands is that it slows down the movement of the exercise from the added resistance when you pull. This allows you to increase muscle mass rather than going too far with the stretches. Going overboard with stretches can also harm tendons and lead to injury. That is why it's important to keep in mind the main purpose when doing yoga exercises, which is to gain strength and improve the overall quality of life and not to reach new limits when stretching.

Yoga has been practiced by human civilization for more than 5000 years. It was first practiced in Northern India and was strongly linked to religion. Indians used yoga as a way to connect with a higher power and increase awareness. In modern days, yoga is a globally widespread practice. It is commonly used among all ages as it is proven to be both physically and mentally beneficial. Older adults who practice yoga were less stressed, had better sleep, and were more physically flexible when compared to adults who didn't include it in their daily life.

According to statistics, the number of Americans over the age of 50 that practiced yoga rose from 4 million in 2012 to more than 14 million in 2016. That is almost 4 times higher. The growth in popularity isn't just a coincidence. The reason yoga practice has reached an all-time high is that people are now starting to realize that the benefits of yoga are more than what was expected.

Another reason why yoga is a great choice for seniors is that it holds a lesser risk of getting injured. Using resistance bands solely for building up muscle takes some time and patience to adapt. Plus, it can be dangerous for beginners. That is why it is recommended to start using resistance bands to first heal the body through rehabilitation exercises, and then slowly start combining it with yoga.

This will gradually help the body heal at its maximum capacity which will allow it to regain double the strength it could have regained by immediately starting to do strengthening exercises. Another thing about yoga is that it is never too late to start, no matter how old you get! (Just make sure to get a doctor's approval before you start including it in your routine.)

Yoga has many life-changing health benefits. One of the benefits older adults like the most about practicing yoga is that it relieves and keeps chronic pain away. The previous chapters informed you on how you can relieve chronic pain. But aging will always do its thing and bring this pain back if you go back to your usual routine. Yoga prevents that. This is because it alleviates the areas where the pain is present.

A study found something unique and new about how chronic pain is connected to stress. The study found that although the pain was due to complications that came with aging, it was highly impacted by the levels of stress a person experienced in their lives.

The area of the body that caused the pain was more inflamed in seniors that had a more stressful life than the ones who didn't. And because yoga has a huge impact on fighting stress levels, it automatically helps reduce inflammation in the painful areas of the body. Typically, statistics show that seniors that start practicing yoga consistently, require less pain medication after around the fourth week.

Yoga also helps with insomnia. Up to 48% of adults over the age of 60 have experienced insomnia symptoms. While 12%-20% of adults suffer from regular insomnia disorder. Surprisingly, yoga has shown to be more effective in soothing levels of insomnia than drinking herbal sleep tea.

There have even been instances that it has been more effective than sleep medication. This is all due to the impact yoga has on your breathing. By practicing your breathing technique with yoga exercises, your breathing automatically slows down. When this happens, your body produces more melatonin, which is a sleep-inducing hormone that is often lacking in adults who experience insomnia symptoms.

The Centers for Disease Control and Prevention highly recommend seniors practice yoga to fight high blood pressure. Also known as "the silent killer" high blood pressure is common in half of the people over the age of 55. But the thing is that many adults are not even aware of having this problem. This is all because in most cases, high blood pressure does not cause any signs of symptoms or illness.

Its effects come suddenly and instantly, usually with a stroke, sudden kidney disease or heart disease, and even vascular dementia. If lifestyle changes are not made to decrease blood pressure then its sudden effects may end up reducing the quality of life. Many seniors have reported having lower blood pressure after their very first day of doing yoga.

The biggest thing that is often overlooked by seniors is stress. Not managing stress levels can cause severe changes to your body. Stress is universally known for speeding up the aging process, making you look older. Seniors that do not manage stress or experience more stress in life experience what is called an internal fight or flight response. When you experience constant high levels of stress your autonomic and endocrine systems in the body will be activated. This leads your body to respond in unregulated ways, which is known as the fight or flight response.

Although it varies from person to person, seniors have a more hidden response to stress than younger adults do. Usually, younger adults respond to stress by lashing out, screaming, shutting down, and avoiding. Seniors on the other hand respond to stress by experiencing frequent headaches, increased blood pressure, shortness of breath, and increased blood sugar just to name a few. Seniors that suffer from dementia also experience high-stress levels that are mostly created by confusion.

Practicing yoga lets you focus more on your breathing which allows more oxygen to enter the bloodstream. As the oxygen levels in your body increase, your heart relaxes and your heartbeat slows down. Higher levels of oxygen in the bloodstream also help in relaxing the tension in the abdomen area where stress pain is usually felt. Focusing on our breathing is also a great way to be in the present moment and practice mindfulness.

Yoga prevents falls and injury. Because yoga is also a muscle strengthening practice, it leads to better stability and balance. It is highly known for strengthening the back muscles and core muscles, which is the primary reason why it can help you with better balance and prevent falls.

Holding a yoga pose for several breaths is a highly efficient way to improve body flexibility. This is because it allows the connective tissues and the muscles to relax. The relaxation of the muscles causes them to loosen up and give you the benefit of increasing your body's range of motion.

Yoga also improves respiration. Lungs do not have any muscle. However, you can still strengthen your lungs to hold more oxygen by practicing yoga. Your lungs fully mature at the age of 25. But, after the age of 35 lungs start deteriorating. This explains why you may experience shortness of breath more frequently as you age. Even though lung deterioration cannot be prevented, it can be slowed down as a process.

What happens as you age is that the Alveoli of the lungs lose their shape through time, which causes them to become baggy. The diaphragm also plays a huge role in shortness of breath. Aging weakens the diaphragm, which causes difficulty when inhaling and exhaling. One study found that women that followed a 3-month yoga program had less trouble breathing and falling short of breath.

Even though yoga offers some amazing benefits for the mind and body, it is always a good idea to talk to your healthcare provider and get professional recommendations before starting yoga. Some adults may not be capable of accomplishing a certain set of yoga exercises due to their medical conditions.

For example, people that suffer from glaucoma, which is an eye condition caused by damage to the optic nerve, should not practice any sort of yoga exercise with their head down. This is because too much blood to the head can increase eye pressure and further damage the optic nerve. Your doctor will give you similar advice if you suffer from any complications or conditions.

The next step to prepare for yoga is to gather all of the gear that is necessary to start your exercises. The first and most important thing to keep in mind before starting any yoga session is to wear loose clothing. Because yoga is tightly connected to breathing exercises, wearing tight clothing can cause unease. It can also impact the effectiveness of the practice as wearing tight clothing doesn't allow your body to fully inhale, leading to lower levels of stress being reduced.

When it comes to shirts, it's best to find a stretchy, light, and fitted top.

You would not want anything too loose as the shirt can end up all in your eyes in case you bend down during a stretch. Legwear is the most complicated, as it might tighten the belly area. Finding legwear that is light on the belly and does not fall when exercised is as rare as gemstones. But it's not impossible to find them! Footwear on the other hand is not needed when practicing yoga as the practice is originally done barefoot. If you would prefer to wear something, then wearing a pair of non-slip socks will do the trick.

Yoga doesn't need any other gear besides the mat, and of course, the resistance bands. When doing more traditional yoga exercises, a yoga mat is crucial. When it comes to choosing a mat, you need one that is as long (if not a bit longer) than you are when you lie down. Also, the material of the mat depends on its price. Although price doesn't necessarily impact the quality of practicing yoga, it does indicate the kind of quality the mat is built from.

Cheap mats are made from PVC while the more expensive ones are made with materials such as cotton, rubber, or jute, which are more environmentally friendly. When choosing the thickness of the mat don't go with anything that is more than half an inch thicker. Thicker yoga mattresses can cause you to lose balance and get injured. Thick mats are also a huge pain when it comes to carrying them around as they are pretty heavy.

The last step to prepare for a yoga session is to always start slowly. Keep in mind that you need to get enough rest between each yoga exercise, especially if you are a beginner. Do not go to the next exercise immediately. Give your body 20-40 seconds to relax in between each exercise.

Also, yoga is not a competition. If you are doing yoga along with your friend, partner, or collectively, remember to do the stretch at your own pace. Practicing yoga is done by doing whatever makes you feel comfortable so you can focus on your breathing and mindfulness.

Another very important thing before starting yoga is knowing that it should never hurt. You might feel a slight burning sensation that comes from the resistance band pulls, but any intense burning or other body pain means that you are unnecessarily pushing yourself too far during the exercise. Whenever you feel that a certain yoga position is causing you pain or discomfort, then focus on other exercises that are easier to complete.

Since every yoga position requires you to also practice breathing techniques, it's important to know how to properly breathe during exercises. You need to first relax the abdomen before inhaling for 3-4 seconds. Do not force yourself to fill up your lungs with as much air as possible when inhaling. The right way to do it is to inhale normally, neither too fast nor too slow, but as much as you feel comfortable. Then immediately exhale slowly, for 6-8 seconds.

There are many types of yoga. All have different focuses. In the following practices, you will be learning some of the best yoga exercises from the easiest exercises to start with up to more traditional exercises. Preparing for yoga is the first step to ensuring that you are doing the practice right.

Here are some easy and highly effective yoga exercises you can start even if you have never practiced it before. The first pose you will want to start with does not include resistance bands. Look at it more as a warm-up and a preparation for the yoga session you are about to do. The exercise is called the tree pose and its main purpose is to strengthen your balance for the upcoming yoga positions. If you are exercising at home you can also use a chair or the wall when performing this position for the first time.

Tree pose

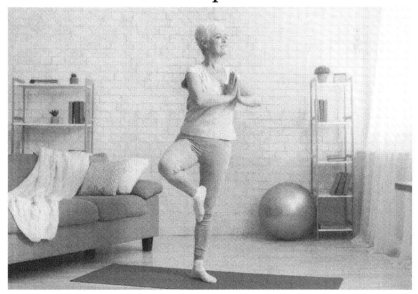

1. Stand up in a straight position
2. Straighten your back and open your chest for air to effortlessly fill your lungs.
3. Stand close to a chair or wall for stability
4. Raise your hands up straight above your head
5. Put one leg on the other leg's calf

6.Do a few breaths while holding the pose

7.Rest for 20-40 seconds before continuing with the other leg

If you find it difficult to maintain balance, then use one hand to hold on to a chair or a wall while continuing to keep the other hand up straight. As you get better at it, remove your hand from the chair or wall for a few seconds to further improve balance. Only do this if you are confident that you can maintain balance by yourself for a few seconds. If you are not confident enough, do not let go of the chair or wall while performing the exercise.

Upper body stretch

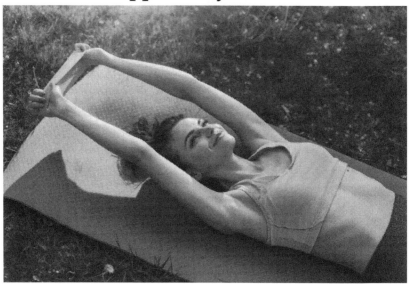

1.Lie down on a yoga mat

2.Hold a short loop band with both hands

3.Keep your back straight and relaxed

4.Keep both arms and legs stretched

5.Maintain position for several breaths

Side bends

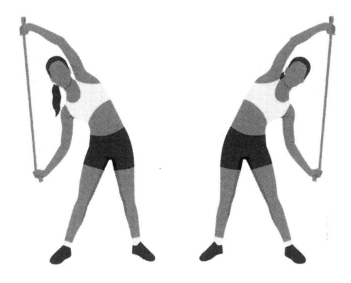

1. Take the thera band and place it above your head
2. Open feet hip-width and stand straight or sit on a chair
3. Keep body straight and relaxed
4. Slowly go down sideways while exhaling and come up inhaling
5. Repeat several times on both sides
6. Rest for 20-40 seconds before switching sides

Keep the head tight when doing the exercise and avoid moving it. Allow it to move along with your body. Make sure you are keeping your hands straight. The only thing that should be moving in this position is your spine. Now, when it comes to the breathing technique, inhale as soon as you bend down. Exhale while coming up in the starting position and inhale again while bending down. Repeat this cycle for a few breaths.

Chest stretch

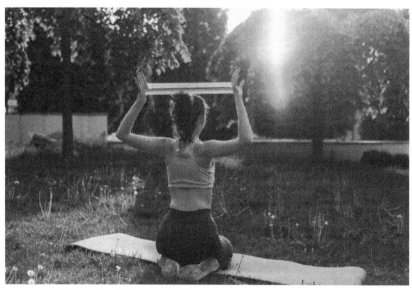

1. Maintain sitting position
2. Hold a thera band or loop band with both hands
3. Make sure your hands are behind your head
4. Keep the band slightly pulled while inhaling and exhaling
5. Maintain position for several breaths

Arm stretch

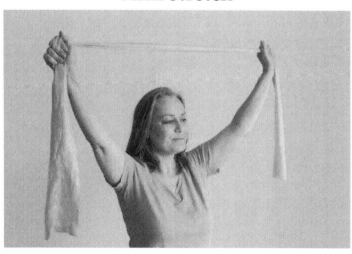

1. Place a short loop band around your wrists

2. Stand straight or sit down straight on a chair

3. Hold both hands in front of you and keep them straightened

4. Keep the band slightly pulled while inhaling and exhaling

5. Repeat for a few breaths until your arms feel fatigued

Close the yoga session by repeating the tree pose used you opened the session with. While holding on to a chair, try to practice the pose with your eyes closed this time. Focus deeply on your breathing and keep your mind in the present moment.

While doing this you can also focus on the feeling of your foot touching the calf, the feeling of your hand holding on to the chair, the outdoor noises, or indoor silence. This final closing practice not only helps with balance but also reduces stress levels, decreases blood pressure, and releases healthy amounts of melatonin hormones.

Chapter 5: Shoulder Exercises

Science has yet to find how to fully prevent the effects that come with age. But nature has given us a solution right in front of our doorsteps, which is the ability to exercise our body anytime and anywhere that we want to. It has always been one of the thousands of medicines that nature has provided us with. Yet, people still take exercising for granted and see it as a chore rather than a privilege that mankind is equipped with.

If you're a senior, you may want to consider strength training as an option for improving your health and fitness. The following chapters will help you determine whether strength training is right for you and how to get started.

Strength training has many benefits, including improved bone density, muscle mass, balance, posture, and lower-back strength. It can also help improve overall body composition by increasing lean muscle mass while decreasing body fat. This means that your body will burn more calories throughout the day—even when you're at rest.

Strength training is also known to reduce risk factors associated with osteoporosis (bone loss), type 2 diabetes, heart disease, high blood pressure, obesity, depression, and anxiety. By adding strength training to your weekly routine, you may be able to reduce or even reverse some of these risk factors in just a few months.

Strength training is one of the best things you can do for your health at any age. It's never too late to start. Studies show that people who start as late as age 60 will see health benefits from strength training. If you've been thinking about starting but haven't yet taken that first step yet, here are some reasons why now is a great time to get started.

In the United States, more than 50 percent of adults over the age of 65 are considered obese or overweight. Obesity increases the risk for type 2 diabetes, heart disease, and other chronic illnesses. Exercise is one of the best ways to maintain a healthy weight and improve your overall health.

It can even delay — or even prevent — many of these diseases from developing in the first place. If you're like most seniors, you've probably heard about how important exercise is for your overall health and well-being. However, many people find it hard to get motivated to start an exercise routine.

Exercising with resistance bands is considered an anaerobic exercise but bands can be dangerous if used improperly. Always use a piece of furniture nearby (like a strong chair or table) while doing exercises that involve standing on your hands or feet. This will give you something to instantly hold on to in case you lose balance.

Don't allow more than one person to hold each side of a resistance band at once unless it is specifically designed for multiple users (such as resistance tubes). You should also use caution with heavy resistance band levels (usually the darker colored bands). If you have fragile wrists or ankles, use caution when using heavy resistance bands because they may cause discomfort or even injure your wrists or ankles due to their extreme nature. Be aware of how much force is being exerted by each band and always be careful when using them. It is recommended to start with light bands and move up to medium level if you are an older adult.

Now, anaerobic exercises are slightly different from both rehab and yoga. Although both rehabilitation of the body and yoga practices are technically considered branches of exercise, they serve more for healing and stretching the body. Anaerobic exercise mostly focuses on gaining strength, and power, burning fat, and training the body to reach new limits.

Sure, all three types of physical activity are strongly tied to one another and have a lot of things in common. For example, all of them are vital for maintaining good mental health, reducing stiffness, and increasing muscle and bone mass and come with a long list of health benefits.

Another key difference between anaerobic exercise is that it does not focus on breathing techniques to gain energy. It involves more intense activities that do not last longer than 1 or 2 minutes. After fully healing from rehab training, and after practicing yoga for a few weeks, your body is likely capable of handling basic anaerobic exercises. It is always best to talk to a medical professional at first.

Weakening of the shoulders due to inactivity can lead to an increased risk of injury such as damage of the muscles and tendons of the rotator cuff. These injuries can happen to any age group, but they are most common in people over 40. A rotator cuff is a group of four muscles that allow you to raise and rotate your arm. It also helps keep the ball of your shoulder joint in its socket.

The most common injury to this area is a tear in the supraspinatus tendon, which passes through the middle of your shoulder and attaches to the top of your arm bone (humerus). The supraspinatus is one of the four muscles that make up the rotator cuff. As its name suggests, it helps lift your shoulder toward your ear and rotate it outward from your body (abduction).

Pain from this type of tear comes on gradually, often after lifting something heavy or repetitive movements such as throwing a ball or swinging a golf club for many years. It may feel like a burning sensation or stiffness when you raise your arm above shoulder level, but there's no swelling or bruising. If left severely untreated, some tears heal on their own with time and rest, but others need surgery to repair them.

Frozen shoulder is another painful condition that makes it difficult to move your shoulder. It occurs when the tissue around the joint becomes stiff and tight. This causes pain and limited motion of the affected shoulder.

There are several theories about how frozen shoulders happen. The most common theory is that it happens when surrounding tissue becomes scarred. This scar tissue then restricts movement in the joint and causes pain when you try to move your arm. Other theories include cartilage degeneration, nerve damage, and muscle imbalance or weakness at the joint.

Frozen shoulders can affect people of all ages, but it most often affects people between 40 and 60 years old. It's also more common in women than men (2:1 ratio). Individuals who have diabetes, thyroid disease, Parkinson's disease, or heart disease are at higher risk for developing frozen shoulders.

People who have had surgery on their shoulders are also more likely to develop this condition because they don't use their arms as much after surgery than before it happened. If you injured your shoulder during an accident or fall and haven't used it much since then, you may develop a frozen shoulder from lack of use over time.

Arthritis is the most common joint disease and affects more than 50 million people in the United States. Arthritis causes pain, stiffness, and swelling of the joints, and can lead to deformity and disability if not properly managed. Arthritis in the shoulder is called shoulder osteoarthritis. It is a type of degenerative arthritis that causes pain and swelling in one or both shoulders.

This condition starts as early as age 50, although it can begin at any age. The first symptom is increasing pain while lifting or rotating your arms. This pain is mostly felt at the shoulder area. You may also experience stiffness after sleeping on one side of your body. As osteoarthritis progresses, painful movement becomes more common, especially during activities that require overhead movements like throwing a ball or lifting heavy objects overhead (such as groceries).

The most common cause of osteoarthritis is overuse. Overuse occurs when your joints are used too much for too long with no rest periods to allow them to recover from injury or stress. A sudden injury may also lead to osteoarthritis if you continue using an injured joint too much before it has healed properly.

Balancing a yoga and strength training routine in your life is extremely crucial if you want to reduce or prevent any of these shoulder conditions. As mentioned previously, the shoulders are one of the largest areas of the body. Because they are the number one mobility provider for the upper body, weakened or damaged shoulders highly impact the quality of life. A great way to start a shoulder strengthening workout is by practicing good posture.

Wall press

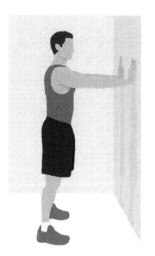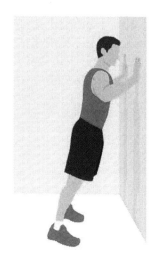

1. Stand up straight against a wall
2. Keep head, neck, shoulders, hip, and heels up against the wall
3. Keep your shoulders straight
4. Make sure your arms are straight and your palms are against the wall
5. Keep your feet closed
6. Keep the posture for 2 minutes while practicing deep breathing

This will straighten the shoulders as well as feed them with a good amount of oxygen to start the shoulder strengthening exercises.

Front raise

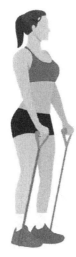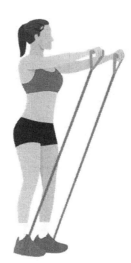

1. Step on a long loop or thera band with both feet
2. Grab the ends of the band with both hands
3. Keep your legs straight and open them shoulder-width
4. Keep shoulders and neck straight and firm
5. Place both hands in front of you at a 90° angle with palms facing down
6. Pull the band upward, fully straightening your arms above your head
7. Slowly go to starting position
8. Repeat 8 times with 3 sets

Lateral raises

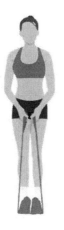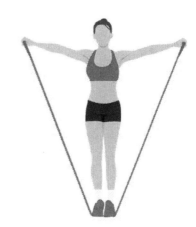

1. Maintain the same position of the front raise exercise
2. Bring your arms to the sides at a 90° angle while holding on to the band
3. Close your legs fully while continuing to keep them straight
4. Pull the thera band above your head in a "Y" position
5. Slowly come back down to starting position
6. Repeat 6-8 times with 3 sets

When doing this exercise, it is not necessary to fully stretch your arms above your head. Take it easy and pull the band over your head as far as you feel comfortable.

One-sided lateral raise

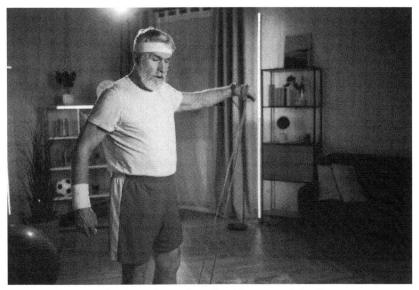

1. Step in the long loop band with your right foot
2. Grab the other end of the band with your right hand
3. Keep your hand straight and on the side with the palm facing down
4. Open legs at shoulder width and keep them straight
5. Keep shoulder and head straight while pulling the band sideways
6. Pull until it reaches shoulder height
7. Repeat 8 times on each side with 2 sets

The shrug pull

SHOULDER SHRUG
WITH RESISTANCE BAND

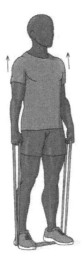 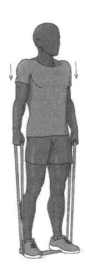

1. Step on a thera band with both feet
2. Keep your legs straight and open them shoulder-width
3. Wrap the ends of the band with both hands until the band is tight and stretched
4. Keep arms down and straight
5. Pull your shoulders up like you are shrugging
6. Lower the shoulders slowly in starting position
7. Repeat 8 times with 3 sets

UPRIGHT ROW

WITH RESISTANCE BAND

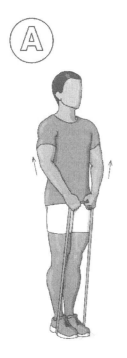

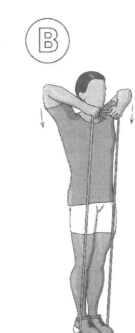

1. Step on a long loop band with both feet
2. Grab the ends of the band with both hands
3. Keep your legs straight and close
4. Put your hands in front of you at pelvic level
5. Pull the band upward until they reach the front of your chin
6. Slowly go to starting position
7. Repeat 8 times with 3 sets

Band dislocates

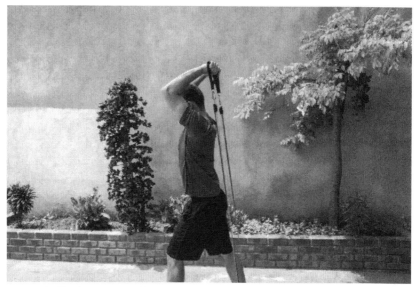

1. Grab your resistance band by both ends and hold it behind your back

2. Keep your arms in a 90° angle above your head

3. Pull the band upwards while slightly lifting your arms in the process

4. During the stretch keep your head and back straight to keep the shoulder blades down

5. Hold this position for approximately 3 seconds

6. Repeat 5-10 times

When you use resistance bands for weight training, the bands have the advantage of stimulating your shoulders just as if you are doing real-world work, such as lifting objects, but without all the dangers that come along with it.

Keep in mind that shoulder strengthening exercises are not recommended to practice if you have chronic or severe shoulder pain. To prevent injury or worsening a condition you may suffer from, you need to get a medical professional's opinion to safely start these shoulder exercises.

Chapter 6: Torso Exercises

The reason why this chapter is called torso and not abdominal exercises is that it's not just what is in front of your body that you need to strengthen, it's also what's around it. By definition, the torso is the trunk of your body. It includes your abdominal muscles, your side muscles, and your back muscles.

The core consists of three layers: anterior (front), lateral (side), and posterior (back). Each layer has its own set of muscles that work together to keep you balanced when standing upright or doing other activities such as walking or bending over to pick something up off the floor. The major muscle groups include:

Rectus abdominis: This is the muscle that makes up the bulk of what people see as a six-pack or a washboard stomach.

External obliques: These muscles run diagonally down each side of your abdomen and are used in side bending and twisting movements.

Internal obliques: Located beneath the external obliques on either side of your abdomen, these muscles assist with rotation and bending, such as when twisting to throw a pitch or swinging a golf club.

Transverse abdominis: This flat muscle sits beneath all other abdominal muscles and wraps around your entire torso like a corset from front to back. It helps stabilize your spine, especially during heavy lifting.

The core — sometimes called the "powerhouse" for its role in generating power and strength — is made up of a complex network of muscles and connective tissues that runs from the base of your skull to the top of your pelvis. This area includes your lower back, hips, abdomen, pelvic floor, and deep hip muscles. Your core is critical for good posture, balance, and movement. It also plays a role in breathing and digestion. Because the core covers such a large area of your body, it has its own chapter in this book. The benefits of strengthening your torso include:

Improved posture. A strong torso helps support the spine and maintain good alignment from head to toe. This reduces strain on ligaments, tendons, and other tissues that support the spine, as well as on joints throughout the body. Stronger abdominal muscles reduce lower back pain by improving posture and reducing back curvature. If you also want to avoid injuries like falling or tripping over objects, you need strong abdominal muscles to support your spine. Stronger spinal muscles will also help you lift heavier objects with greater ease, which reduces the strain on other parts of your body such as your arms and legs.

Better balance and coordination. Stronger muscles help you maintain balance when you're standing still or moving quickly; they also improve coordination between different muscle groups used in movement (such as walking or running). Whether you're lifting something heavy or bending over to tie your shoes, a strong torso will help you perform better in your daily activities.

Better athletic performance. Strengthening your torso also helps you perform better during sports that require quick bursts of energy such as tennis or golf (it can also help prevent injury during such sports). Stronger abdominals may help improve athletic performance by increasing power output from the legs during sprinting or jumping movements.

Relieved pain from sciatica and back injuries. A strong torso can help reduce pressure on nerves in the lower back caused by disc herniation or spinal stenosis (narrowing). This may relieve sciatica-type pain that shoots down the leg. A strong torso also helps stabilize the spine after surgery or injury, which may reduce pain and increase mobility during recovery.

More energy for everyday activities. Many of us spend our days sitting at desks or hunched over computers, which can lead to fatigue or back pain when we try to stand up straight again. By strengthening your core muscles, you'll feel more energized so that you can do everyday tasks without getting tired as fast!

You can strengthen your core through exercises such as planks and crunches. Planks are great exercises to strengthen the back and abdominal muscles. They also improve posture and balance, and they help prevent back pain. To do a plank, lie face down on the floor on your elbows and toes (make sure to wear shoes), holding yourself up in a straight line from head to heels.

Hold this position for as long as possible without letting your hips sag or your lower back arch. If you can't hold this position for 30 seconds, try holding it for 10 seconds at first and increase your time gradually over time until you're able to hold it for 30 seconds without allowing any sagging or arching in your back or hips. If this still seems like a challenge, then place both knees on the ground and continue to perform the plank. You can slowly upgrade to a regular plank once you feel more confident or after having gained more strength by exercising regularly.

Crunches help build abdominal strength by exercising the rectus abdominis muscle — the "six-pack" muscle that runs down the front of your abdomen — along with other muscles in your back and hips. While crunches are an effective way to strengthen these muscles, they don't necessarily improve overall function or mobility in daily life.

For example, if you have poor posture or weak hips or glutes (buttocks), then these imbalances may contribute to poor movement patterns that can lead to lower back pain over time. The best way to fix this is by adding resistance bands to your torso strengthening exercises. Here are a list of torso strengthening exercise you can perform:

Torso: Chest

Chest press

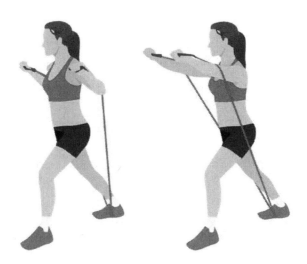

1. Step on a long loop band or tube band with one foot
2. Place the other foot forward and bend it slightly
3. Grab the other end of the loop band (the band should be behind you)
4. Pull by moving your arms in front of your chest
5. Go back to the starting position (arms should not go behind your back. Keep them parallel with your shoulders)
6. Repeat 6 times for each leg

Chest crossover

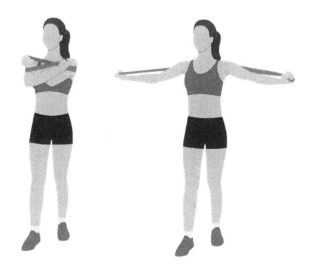

1.Place a thera band around your back

2.Grab each side of the band with its corresponding hand

3.Straighten your arms

4.Keep your back straight and your neck gently tucked

5.Cross your arms in front of your chest

6.Repeat for 8-10 reps

Torso: Upper Abdomen

Cobra stretch

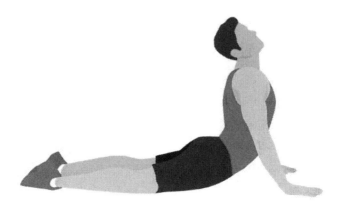

1. Lie face down on your yoga mat
2. Keep your legs straight
3. Slowly raise your body up while curing your back
4. Keep shoulders straight
5. Maintain the position for 20 seconds while breathing normally

Alternate heel touches

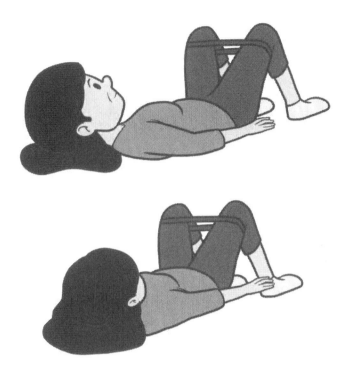

1. Lie down on the yoga mat
2. Keep legs bent with the sole on the ground
3. Keep arms straight
4. Slightly raise your head in a semi-crunch position
5. Move your core from the side
6. While moving pretend as if you are trying to reach your feet with your arms
7. Repeat for 10 reps

Torso: Mid-back muscles

Overhead pull

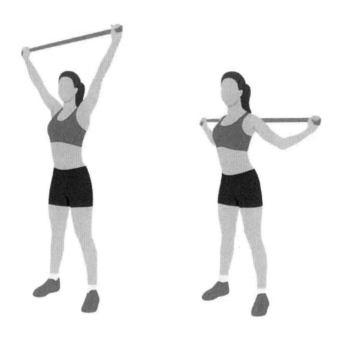

1. Stand in a vertical position
2. Grab a band on both sides with each hand
3. Position the band over your head
4. Pull the band outward while bringing it down to your back
5. Repeat for 6-8 reps

Chapter 7: Arm Exercises

The arms are an important part of the body and can be used as a gauge for overall fitness. If you have weak arms, there is a good chance that you will also have weak legs and a weak back. Strong arms allow you to keep yourself in good shape for years to come. A strong set of arms makes it possible for you to lift heavy items with ease, do more push-ups and pull-ups, throw objects farther, swing harder at golf, etc.

A lot of people think that you can only get healthy arms by lifting heavy weights. But the truth is, you can also get toned and shapely arms by working out using only resistance banks. Hands down, the best way to build strong, toned arms is strength training. When you work out your muscles, they get bigger and stronger to handle the stress of being used. As a result, they grow.

In addition to arm-related exercises, there are many other ways that you can strengthen your arms. For example, if you want to improve your grip strength or make it easier on yourself when lifting heavy items such as groceries or suitcases into the car trunk or onto the top shelf of your closet... try using short loop bands around your wrists and elbows when training! Exercising your arms with bands has a series of health benefits which include:

Improved posture: We often think of posture as being something that only affects our appearance but in fact, it affects our physical health too. A poor posture can cause pain in the neck and shoulders, which can lead to headaches and back pain. Exercising your arms will help to build up the muscles in the area so that they are better equipped to support your body weight when you walk upright.

Better balance: The muscles in your arms help maintain balance when standing or walking on uneven surfaces because they provide stability for your body weight. Therefore, exercising these muscles will help improve their strength which will make it easier for you to perform other movements throughout your day. In addition, a stronger upper body means that you will have more control over your movements and be less likely to fall over if you trip or slip. This is especially important as we get older when our balance becomes less stable than it was when we were younger.

Reduced risk of injury: Stronger arm muscles protect us from injury by helping us perform everyday tasks more easily without straining our joints or tendons too much. This allows us to enjoy life without pain or discomfort!

Muscle Tone: Stronger muscles help you maintain a more active lifestyle because they support your body weight better than weak muscles do. When you have strong muscles, they help you to burn calories more quickly throughout the day due to their increased metabolism rate. A combination of strength training arm exercises with aerobic exercises will help you achieve this goal.

Bone Health: As you get older, your bones start to lose their density. This is a natural part of the aging process, but it can be slowed down by strength training. Studies show that those who lift weights tend to lose less bone mass than those who don't. By placing a reasonable amount of stress on your bones, resistance band training can build bone density, which is especially important in later years of life. This in turn can even reduce your risk of developing diseases such as osteoporosis.

Arm strength is a very common term in the world of fitness. It's typically used to refer to how much you can lift or push, but it also refers to how many reps you can do before reaching failure, and how long you can hold something at all. Arm strength is important for almost any activity you can imagine — from driving a car to typing on a computer. The stronger your arms are, the more stable they will be, and the more weight they can hold without fatiguing as quickly.

For your upper arms, there are two primary muscles that you likely know well; the biceps, the triceps and forearms. Biceps consists of two heads: biceps brachii (long head) and biceps brachialis (short head). Both heads work together during elbow flexion and shoulder adduction however the short head is more involved during shoulder extension while both heads are active during pronation/supination (rotating forearm). The biceps brachialis is located on the underside of the upper arm so it's important to train this area.

The triceps make up over two-thirds of the upper arm and are responsible for pushing movements such as bench presses and dips. They are best worked with compound exercises like push-ups but can also be trained by isolation exercises like push-downs.

Forearm muscles. Other than that, there's one often overlooked feature of our arms, even though it makes up for about half of them; our forearms. These are often neglected, but we use them in nearly every functional movement you can name. The forearms are a complex network of muscles, tendons, and ligaments that help us grasp objects and stabilize our wrists for many movements. They're also one of the most neglected areas in the gym, with most people focusing on biceps and triceps instead.

Forearm workouts are a great way to tone your arms. Your forearms are the muscles on the outside of your arm from your elbow to your wrist. They help you pinch, grasp and lift items with more weight than you can manage with just your hands alone. You may want to take a few minutes before exercising to stretch out your wrists, fingers, and forearms so that you do not strain any muscles during exercise.

Forearm workouts are an effective way to build strength and endurance in your hands and arms. They are also a great way to increase hand strength so you can play sports more effectively. Forearm exercises can be done at home with a variety of tools, including hand grippers and wrist weights. You can also do these exercises using your body weight as resistance. There are many ways to strengthen your forearms through exercise, including:

Wrist curls - This is one of the most basic forearm exercises. You simply lift small weights with your wrists, holding the weights close to your body so that only your wrist moves up and down as you curl them up toward your chest then lower them back down again.

Static holds - Static holds work by forcing you to hold on to an object for as long as possible without letting go. For example, try holding onto a barbell or dumbbells with straight arms for 1 minute at a time until you feel like you cannot hold on any longer.

One common way of measuring grip strength is by using a dynamometer (also known as a handgrip dynamometer). You squeeze the handle with all your might until it stops moving; then the device calculates how much force you applied during that period and displays it in pounds or kilograms.

Seniors tend to lose strength in their upper body primarily because they do not strengthen this area as much as other areas, such as the lower body or core area. The loss of muscle mass in your arms can put you at risk for falls because there is less support for your body weight when reaching out. This is why it is important to exercise these areas regularly.

You should exercise your arms at least twice a week. In general, aim for two to three strength-training sessions per week. You could do this by splitting up your workouts into two sessions or by doing one longer session each week. Strength training is important for everyone, but it's especially important for people who want to increase their muscle mass.

If you're new to strength training, start slowly with one or two days per week of exercising your arms. As you get stronger and more comfortable with the exercises, add another day of arm workouts every few weeks until you're up to two or three days per week. Your healthcare provider will be able to design a program for you that meets your needs and goals. Always consult a doctor before starting an exercise program or diet.

When it comes to resistance band exercises for arms, dumbbells are usually the go-to option for most people because they're relatively cheap and easy to store in your home gym closet or under your bed. While dumbbells do have their advantages — namely that they don't roll away when you lay them down — they also have some drawbacks such as being bulky when storing them at home (they take up a lot of space).

Resistance bands on the other hand offer an excellent alternative that is cheaper than traditional dumbbells and takes up less space than free weights. These are 5 great arm exercises you can practice while using resistance bands:

Arm pulls

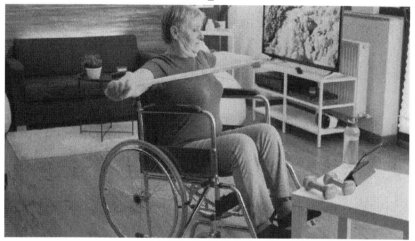

1. Grab your resistance band by both ends and hold it in front of your chest
2. Keep your arms straight with your palms facing down
3. Pull the band sideways
4. During the stretch keep your head and back straight
5. Hold this position for approximately 3 seconds
6. Repeat 5-10 times with 2 sets

Wrist Pulls

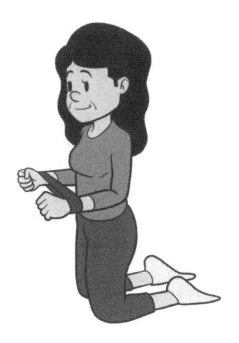

1.Place a short loop band around your wrists
2.Keep your arms in front of you at a 90° angle
3.Keep your back and shoulders straight
4.Pull your arms out
5.Go back to starting position
6.Repcat for 5-8 rcps

Y raise

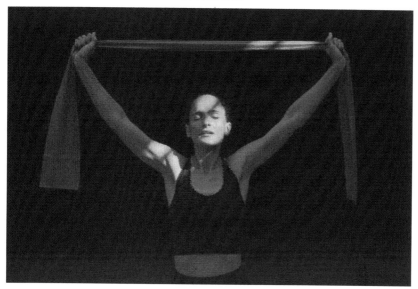

1. Take a long loop or tube band and raise it above your head
2. Keep your back straight and your neck gently tucked
3. Keep your arms straight in a "Y" position
4. Pull the band in both hands until the "Y" is slightly wider
5. Go back to starting position
6. Repeat for 5-8 reps

Side lifts

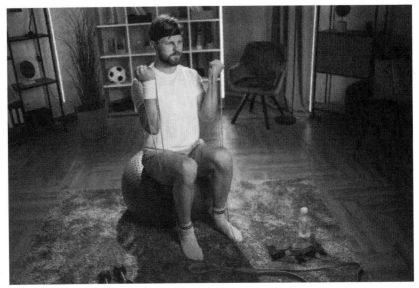

1. Sit down on a chair and place both feet on top of a thera band
2. Grab each side of the band with its corresponding hand
3. Keep arms slightly bent
4. Raise your arms sideways
5. Go back to resting position
6. Repeat for 8-10 reps

Forward pulls

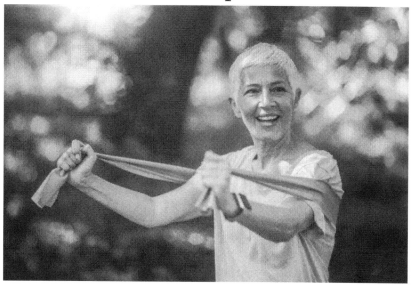

1. Place a thera band around your back
2. Grab each side of the band with its corresponding hand
3. Keep your back straight and your neck gently tucked
4. Keep arms facing up at a 90° angle
5. Pull your hands in front of you until slightly bent
6. Slowly come back to starting position
7. Repeat for 8-10 reps

Arm pullback

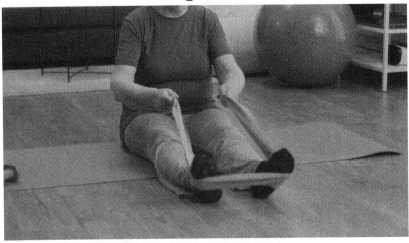

1.Sit on a mat with legs straightened fully

2.Place thera band around your feet and Grab each side of the band with its corresponding hand

3.Keep your legs slightly open and your back straight

4.Keep arms in front of you at a 90° angle

5.Pull band while still keeping your arms at a 90° angle

6.Return to starting position

7.Repeat 8-10 reps

Chapter 8: Leg Exercises

The legs are the largest muscle group in the body, and they're made up of three main muscles — the quadriceps, hamstrings, and glutes. When you work your legs, you are using the largest muscles in your body. This can help you burn a ton of calories and build muscle.

If you want to get fit and stay healthy, it's important to include leg workouts as part of your exercise routine. Leg exercises are an important part of any exercise program, as they help to strengthen your lower body, improve balance and stability, and help to prevent injury.

Leg workouts are often neglected in favor of upper-body workouts, but this is a mistake. Your legs play an important role in helping to support your body weight and reduce the strain on your back and spine.

It's important to maintain strong leg muscles for everyday activities like walking upstairs or getting out of a chair without causing pain or injury. In addition, leg strength helps you perform better in sports that require running or jumping.

The muscles in your lower body are used every time you move your upper body. For example, when you walk or run on the treadmill, you are using all of the muscles in your lower body. When it comes to leg workouts, there are two main types: lower body and upper body. Lower body exercises focus on the muscles surrounding the hip, pelvis, knees, and ankles; these include squats, lunges, and calf raises.

If you have a sedentary lifestyle or suffer from arthritis or other joint pain, leg workouts may be difficult at first. But once you start exercising regularly, your body will adapt and become stronger than it was before.Here are some of the benefits of leg workouts:

Your body needs strong legs if you want to avoid injuries like knee pain or shin splints. Leg workouts can help improve your posture and balance by strengthening your core muscles around your hips and pelvis. These muscles help support the spine so that it doesn't collapse forward under stress (such as when lifting heavy objects). Strengthening them will also improve your overall stability.

Leg workouts are also easier to recover from than upper body workouts because you're using less weight and fewer reps per set. They don't take as much out of your central nervous system as upper body workouts do because you're not pulling the resistance band as much on each set. Here are some reasons why you shouldn't skip leg day:

Improved balance

The legs work together with other muscles in the body to keep us standing up straight and moving forward. This coordination is important for daily activities such as walking or running, but it also helps us perform all types of physical activities like sports or dance. Stronger legs allow us to jump higher and throw farther than people who don't work out their legs regularly!

Build Strength

Leg workouts help build strength in the lower body by working for multiple muscle groups at once in an efficient manner. This includes hamstrings (back of thigh), quadriceps (front of thigh), glutes (buttocks), calves (lower leg), and core muscles like abs and back muscles as stabilizers during exercise movements like squats or lunges for example.

Help prevent osteoporosis

This condition makes it more likely for someone to break a bone. When you work out your legs, this improves the strength of your bones by increasing the amount of density in them. As you age, your body loses more density than it did when you were younger so this is especially important for seniors who are at risk for osteoporosis.

Better Sleep

Leg exercises also help you to sleep better at night because they improve circulation throughout your body. This improves blood flow to your brain so that you can fall asleep faster, stay asleep longer, and wake up feeling more refreshed each morning.

When it comes to exercises, squats are the most rewarding exercises you can do for your lower body — especially if you want strong glutes and thighs! If you've never done squats before but want to start incorporating them into your workout routine, here are a few reasons why they're worth giving a try:

They help build muscle. Squats involve working for multiple large muscle groups at once, which means they're great for building strength and mass. One study found that doing squats for 15 minutes at a fast pace could burn up to 300 calories!

They're easy to incorporate into your routine. You don't have to go to the gym or buy expensive equipment — all you need is an open space and some good music!

If you've never done squats before but want to start incorporating them into your workout routine, here are some of their benefits:

1) Squats help build strong, lean and toned legs.

2) They're a full-body exercise that engages your core, shoulders, and arms along with your lower body.

3) Squats can improve your posture and strengthen your back muscles so you're less likely to develop lower back pain as you age.

4) They improve balance and coordination as well as flexibility in your hips and ankles, which can help prevent injuries while exercising or playing sports.

A few tips to help you improve your leg strength:

Wear compression leggings. Doing so can improve circulation for some people by applying pressure on their legs. This promotes blood flow and supports muscle repair after doing exercises that tone the legs.

Get up from a seated position slowly, especially if you have bad knees or arthritis. If you need help standing up, use a chair or table to assist you with getting up from a seated position. Avoid jumping up to prevent putting too much pressure on your joints. Once you're standing, take at least two steps before sitting back down again — this helps prevent blood pooling in your lower body while sitting down, which can cause clots that lead to deep vein thrombosis (DVT).

Wear shoes that have good arch support and cushioning in the heel. This will help reduce foot pain and fatigue, which can affect your ability to exercise properly.

Start with the lightest bands when doing the exercises as a beginner. Adding too much resistance puts more stress on your muscles and joints than lighter ones do — especially if you haven't used resistance bands before — which can make you feel soreness longer after exercising than if you were using lighter bands.

Rest between sets and workouts so that muscles can recover from being stretched out during exercise sessions. Resting is especially important for people who are new to working out because their bodies need time to strengthen.

When you have a rest day between training sessions, the muscles get stronger as they recover. But if you skip too many workouts in a row, they won't get that chance — and they can start to atrophy instead. It isn't just about losing muscle mass either — if your muscles are too weak when they come back into play again, they could be injured during exercise or in everyday life.

The amount of time between sets is important for building muscle and avoiding injury. When you use resistance bands, your leg fibers tear slightly (this is called microtrauma) and then repair themselves during the rest period between sets. If you don't give yourself enough time for recovery, you risk overtraining and injuring your legs.

Researchers have found that it takes at least 24 hours to 36 hours of rest after working out before your body will respond well to another workout. So if you're strength training two days in a row, there should be at least 48 hours between them. It's also important for beginners to give their bodies an extra day off every week because they recover from exercise more slowly than those who have more experience.

These lower body exercises have been shown to improve balance and stability in seniors who perform them regularly.

Square dance

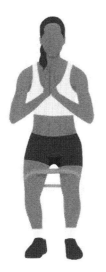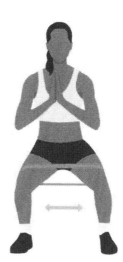

1. Put a short loop band right above the knee
2. Bend knees and open them hip-width while proceeding to stand up straight
3. Place hands on the hips or in front of you
4. Take a step backward with one food and bring the other foot back right after
5. Bring one foot forward and then the other foot forward right after
6. Repeat back and forth several times

For maximum performance try to keep both feet straight and prevent them from turning to the sides too much. It's okay if your feet turn slightly to the side as it is normal for movement. When doing the exercise try to imagine following a square shape when moving your legs back and forth. It is best to do this exercise using two loop bands, one above the knees and one above the ankles. If you do have spare bands lying around then trying this position with two bands will better strengthen your leg area.

Calf pulls

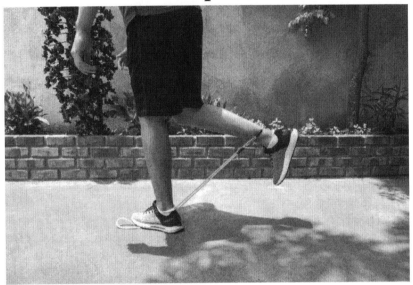

1. Hang on to a chair or a wall for balance
2. Step on one side of a short loop band
3. Place the other leg inside the other end of the loop band
4. Pull the leg upward
5. Slowly go to starting position
6. Repeat for 8-10 reps

Sideway leg raises

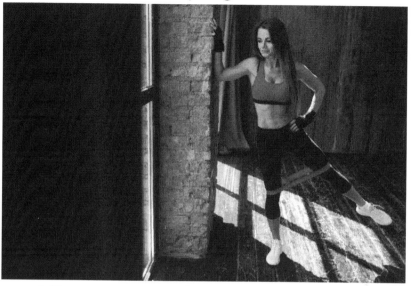

1. Place your arm up against a wall for balance
2. Place a short loop band slightly above ankle level
3. Raise one leg sideways while keeping it straightened out
4. Keep the position for 1 second before returning leg back to the floor
5. Repeat 6-8 times for each leg

Backward leg raises

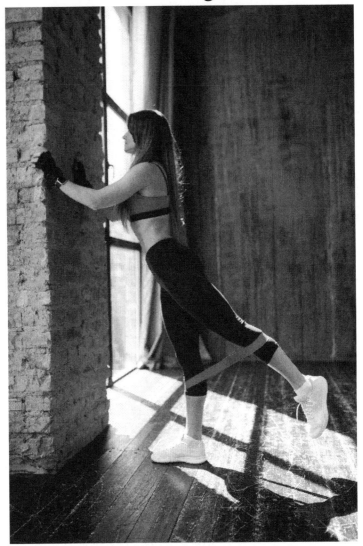

1. Place both arms up against the wall for balance
2. Place a short loop band slightly above ankle level
3. Pull one leg back while keeping it straightened out
4. Keep the position for 1-3 seconds before returning leg on the floor
5. Repeat 6-8 times for each leg

Front crab pulls

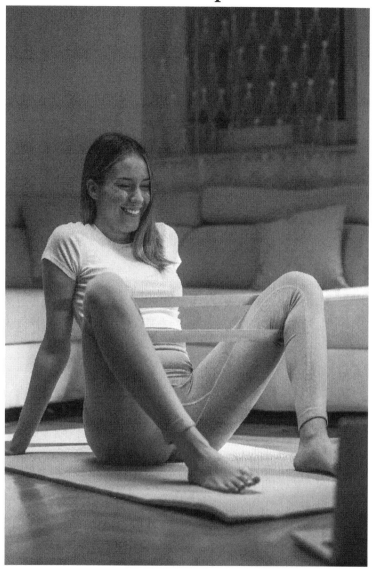

1.Place a short loop band above your knee area

2.Sit down on a yoga mat with legs open at shoulder level

3.Slowly pull sideways with your knees

4.Return to starting position

5.Do 8-10 reps

Side crab pulls

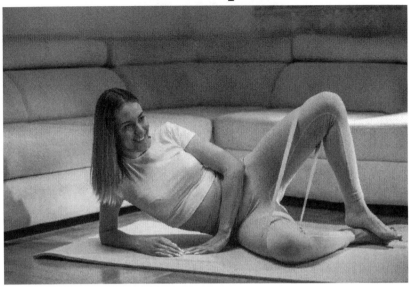

1. Keep the short loop band above your knee area
2. Sit down **_SIDEWAYS_** on a yoga mat with legs open at shoulder level
3. Slowly raise your leg sideways
4. Return to starting position
5. Do 8-10 reps for each leg

Leg raise

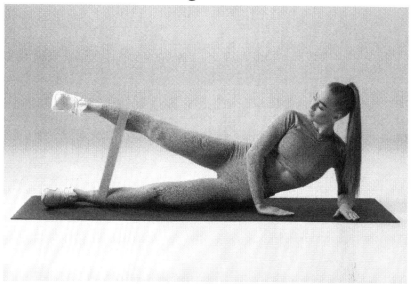

1.Place the short loop band above your ankle area

2.Laydown on a yoga mat with legs fully stretched out

3.Raise leg until you feel resistance (no need to go overboard)

4.Return to starting position

5.Do 8-10 reps for each leg

Chapter 9: Core Work

A strong core is the foundation of a strong body. It's the center of your body, where all movement comes from, and where your power comes from. A strong core helps you maintain good posture while standing or sitting, which leads to better balance. This means less risk of injury during physical activity. It also improves your body mechanics when performing tasks like climbing stairs.

The core includes the lower back, abdomen, and hips (the pelvis). The muscles that make up the core are deep abdominal muscles that stabilize and support the spine, as well as major hip and leg muscles that help with stability and balance.

The core muscles are the main component of a strong core, but other muscles such as the glutes can play a role too. The glutes provide support for your lower back and pelvis, so if those muscles are weak or underdeveloped, it can affect your posture and stability.

Training your core will help improve your overall athleticism and reduce risk factors associated with heart disease, diabetes, and obesity — all of which have been linked to poor muscle tone in this area — according to research published in Medicine & Science in Sports & Exercise in 2010.

In addition to helping improve movement, your core muscles also play an important role in supporting your spine and protecting against back pain. As you age, you may experience some degeneration of these muscles — particularly if you have poor posture or spend long periods sitting at a desk or driving — which can lead to pain and loss of mobility later on.

The core consists of four muscles. These muscles are responsible for trunk stability, spinal mobility, and rotation as well as pelvic stability. They are often referred to as "your belly muscles" because they run around your waistline like a belt that cinches you in tightly from front to back.

These muscles compress the abdomen thus helping to stabilize the lumbar spine during movement by increasing intra-abdominal pressure (pressure inside your abdominal cavity). They also help decrease intra-abdominal pressure during exhalation which allows us to breathe more deeply, promotes proper posture, and supports the proper alignment of our vertebral column during movement.

When these four muscles contract together they allow us to suck in our belly button, lift our rib cage off our pelvis when we inhale, and keep our spine stable while moving our trunk or pelvis in all planes of motion. The deep core muscles have a unique function that is different from other muscles in our body.

They are not meant to move or flex but rather to stabilize the spine and pelvis during the movement of other muscle groups. When we perform exercises such as strengthening exercises, we focus on strengthening these deep core muscles through various movements such as rolls, crunches, side bends, and planks. Strengthening your core has a list of benefits:

Improves flexibility

"The core is the center of stability for our body," says Nicole Albertson, a certified personal trainer and exercise physiologist at the Cleveland Clinic. "If we're not strong in our core, then every time we move, we're going to be relying on our extremities." That means if your core is weak, you'll have to use more energy to move around and pick up objects like groceries and laundry baskets. Plus, you'll have less control over your movements and you will be more likely to injure yourself when lifting weights.

"If you don't engage your core muscles properly while lifting weights or doing resistance exercises (like squats or pushups), then you won't get as much benefit from them," says Albertson. And that means your other muscles won't get as strong either—and neither will the rest of your body!

Increased lifespan

A strong core also helps you live longer. According to the American Council on Exercise (ACE), having a strong core can reduce your risk of chronic diseases such as diabetes, cardiovascular disease, and some cancers. A study published in the Journal of Sports Medicine and Physical Fitness found that core training can reduce your risk of heart disease by lowering blood pressure and improving cholesterol levels. In addition, core training has been shown to improve balance and reduce falls among older adults.

Researchers have also found that a strong core can help prevent osteoporosis by strengthening bones and improving posture. Another study published in the Journal of Strength & Conditioning Research found that women who performed exercises targeting their core had higher bone density than those who didn't.

"We know there's an association between low back pain and decreased physical activity," says Dr. Allison Cieslinski, an orthopedic surgeon at Rush University Medical Center in Chicago. "If you're not moving around enough or doing core exercise, then it's easier for things like arthritis to set in."

Increase stability when participating in sports or other physical activities

A strong core helps you maintain good posture while standing or sitting, which leads to better balance. This means less risk of injury during physical activity such as running. Having a strong core gives you increased functional strength and endurance, which means being able to perform everyday tasks more easily.

Avoid back pain

Core training strengthens the muscles in the abdomen, back, and pelvic floor, which supports the spine and aligns your pelvis in a neutral position so it isn't forced into an anterior tilt (forward tilt). This keeps pressure off the discs between each vertebra, which helps prevent bulging discs from pressing on nerves or causing sciatica pain down your leg.

Ability to breathe easier

The diaphragm is the main muscle for breathing, but if it isn't strong enough to do its job well, you may experience shortness of breath or have trouble sleeping at night because of poor sleep posture (if you're lying on your stomach). Strengthening your core improves diaphragmatic function so you can take deeper breaths without straining yourself.

Have better sexual intercourse

Having a strong core is essential for having good sexual drive! Men who have low testosterone levels may find it difficult to get erections or sustain them during sexual activity if they don't have a strong core. Women may find that they're unable to reach climax unless they have a tight abdominal wall and pelvic floor muscles that contract during these climaxes. A weak core may also cause lower back pain during intercourse due to poor biomechanics or alignment issues such as lordosis (swayback).

But what happens when you have a back injury? Or if you're older and have been living your life sitting down all day long? The answer is that these deep core muscles become inhibited or dysfunctional due to inflammation or poor motor control from years of living an unbalanced lifestyle (i.e., sitting too much). In this case, instead of strengthening these muscles as intended with Pilates or yoga moves, you need to inhibit them further by performing exercises that require too much movement in one direction (i.e., flexion) instead of stabilization.

To understand why these muscles are important for trunk control, we must first review how they work together. When you see a person bend over and touch their toes (without bending at the hips), they will likely have an exaggerated inward curve in their low back (lordosis). This is due to their weak deep core muscles allowing excessive arching of their spine during this movement task.

The deep core muscles also act as a natural shock absorber for your spine. The more toned and strong these muscles are, the better they can support your spine's curvature and keep it upright when you bend over, lift something heavy or jump up on a high step. They also help to prevent back pain by providing support for your back when you stand up straight or bend forward at the waist.

When these muscles become weak or injured they can cause low back pain, SI joint dysfunction (pain), hip issues such as hip bursitis or labral tears, knee pain due to patellar tendonitis (jumper's knee), groin strains/strains/pulls/tears, hamstring strains/strains/pulls/tears and even shoulder impingement syndrome. The best way to keep your body strong and healthy is to perform core exercises at least three times a week. These workouts can be done anytime and anywhere.

Planks are a great way to strengthen your core and improve balance, but they can be challenging. If you're new to planks, start with a knee plank (you'll need a yoga mat or some carpeting) before working up to the full version. "Even if you're in good shape, this exercise can be tough," says Heather Turgeon, an exercise physiologist at the University of New Hampshire. "That's why it's important to build up slowly."

"Planks are one of the best exercises to strengthen your core," says Grant Cohn, owner of Peak Performance Fitness in New York City. "They work on your entire body — all the muscles that stabilize your spine."

The plank is just a static hold in any position that keeps your back straight and your body in a straight line from head to toes. It's a simple exercise, but it requires a lot of focus and concentration. Aside from planks, there are many other core strengthening exercises you can practice while using resistance bands.

Static squat

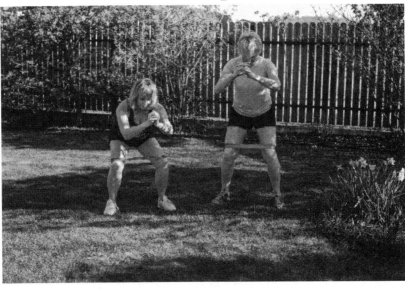

1.Place a short loop band above your knee area

2.Open legs shoulder length

3.Keep back and shoulders straight

4.Take a squat position

5.Make sure your knees don't go in front of your toes

6.Stay in this position for 30 seconds

Russian twists

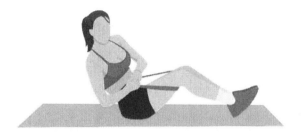

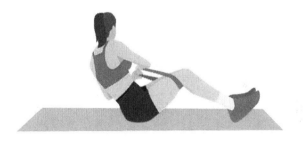

1.Sit on a yoga mat

2.Place a short loop band above your knee area

3.Bend your knees and sit at a 120° angle

4.Keep your feet pointing to the air with your heels touching the ground

5.Grab the band with both hands and twist

6.Twist the body for 15 reps

Core lift

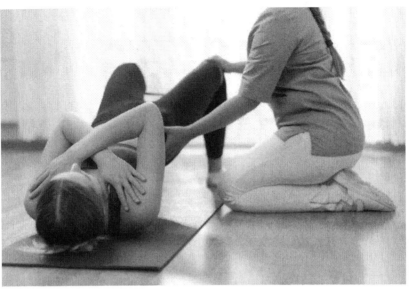

1. Lie down on a yoga mat
2. Place a short loop band above your knee area
3. Keep both arms crossed in front of your chest
4. Move your pelvic area slowly to the top (exhale)
5. Move your pelvic area slowly to the bottom (inhale)
6. Repeat this for 10-15 reps

Side pulls

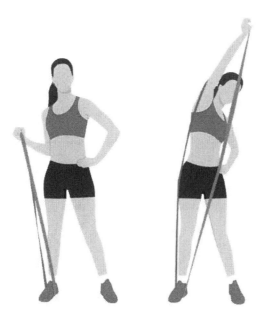

1. Use a long loop band or long thera band
2. Step on one side of the band with one leg and grab the other end with its corresponding hand
3. Keep the same hand with palm facing up and at a 90° angle
4. Raise this hand in a diagonal motion stretching your side core
5. Do this for 8-10 reps for each arm

Abdominal twist

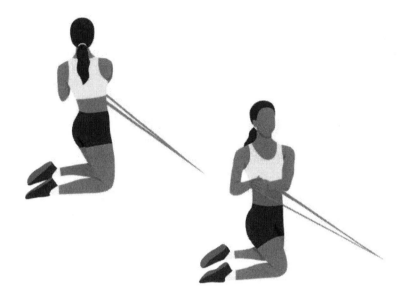

1. Place your resistance band under heavy furniture (table leg)
2. Sit with your knees on the floor and keep the other part of the body straight
3. Grab the other side of the band with both hands
4. Twist your hands along with your core from one side to the other
5. Twist the body for 15 reps

Chapter 10: Moving Forward

There is one crucial element to making a workout effective. This is matching the muscle groups that are being worked. It's not a pretty sight when you're working on your pecs and your shoulders get more of a workout than your chest.

When you're pairing your muscles, you want to make sure that the exercise is taxing them evenly. For example, when pairing your legs with your shoulders, you may wish to do more leg exercises as it's easier for this muscle group to bear more weight than the other. Pairing muscles prevent such a thing from happening.

Pairing muscles is also considered splitting. A split workout is a routine that divides your body into sections, typically upper and lower. Each section of your body is worked on separately, with short rest periods between exercises. Split workouts allow you to focus on one area of the body each day. This can be particularly useful if you want to lose fat while building muscle. There are many ways to structure a split workout, but the most common include:

Full Body Workout - A full body workout trains all of the major muscle groups in a single session. If you are a beginner, then it is recommended only to stick to a full-body workout routine instead of splitting. A splitting workout should be considered only after 6-8 weeks of consistent workout.

A full body workout can be done 2-3 times per week with an emphasis on compound exercises that work multiple muscles at once. Full body workouts are generally performed with lower reps with light to medium resistance and difficulty in order to promote more strength gains than hypertrophy gains.

Upper/Lower Split - An upper/lower split divides your training into two sessions per week where one day focuses primarily on upper body exercises like arms and shoulders, while the other day focuses primarily on lower body exercises such as legs and core. This split allows you to focus more time on each area of your body without fatiguing yourself too much during one session

Push/Pull Split - The push/pull workout splits your body into two parts: pushing muscles and pulling muscles. For example, shoulder day is considered a pushing workout while the core day is considered a pulling workout. This type of split works well because it allows you to work

opposing muscle groups together so you don't get fatigued before your next training session.

Pairing your muscles isn't just about getting more out of your workout; it can also help prevent injury. When you pair large muscle groups together with small ones (for instance, pairing core with arms), you're less likely to over-exert yourself or put too much stress on any one muscle group without giving it enough time to rest between sets. Here is how you can pair muscles during a workout:

Torso (back and chest): These two muscle groups are often paired together because they require similar movement patterns and they both use large amounts of energy during each rep. Some people find it easier to get one workout done in less time by doing these exercises together.

Legs and Arms: The quadriceps (front of the thigh) and hamstrings (back of the thigh) are also best paired together. This is because both are used to produce force during exercise, although they have different functions. For example, the quadriceps work with your glutes to extend your leg forward from a bent position (i.e., knee extension), while the hamstrings pull your leg backward from a straightened position (i.e., knee flexion). Since these movements involve opposing muscle groups working together, you can think of them as a pair that should be worked out at the same time or close together to avoid overtraining or possible injury.

Shoulders and upper torso (chest): Shoulders and upper torso exercises have a lot in common — many of them require you to raise your arms above your head or forward from your body. The front side of your body is generally worked more during chest exercises, while the back side is worked more during shoulder exercises. However, many chest exercises will involve some sort of pushing motion for the shoulders and vice versa.

Back/Biceps: This pairing is a classic weight training combination because these two muscle groups work together during many different exercises such as pull-ups or chin-ups and bicep curls. It's not only possible but also recommended that you pair back exercises with biceps exercises when building muscle mass in this area. This is because when you do a biceps curl or row, you'll be using some of the muscles in your back as well.

Resting

When you work out, your muscle fibers become damaged and sore. Your body needs time to repair this damage, so it can strengthen the muscles and prevent future injuries. If you don't give your body this time to recover, you could end up overtraining and injuring yourself or even wearing down your muscles so much that they stop functioning properly.

Rest days are important for mental health as well. Exercise helps relieve stress by releasing endorphins into the bloodstream, but if you never take time off, this can lead to burnout and even depression. Rest days also give your mind a chance to relax and recharge so that it's ready for another workout session later on.

On rest days, you should still get some physical activity — such as walking or stretching — but avoid strenuous exercise or other activities that would be stressful on your body. You should also take care not to overexert yourself on your rest days; otherwise, you risk getting injured or overtrained.

The purpose of resting is to give your body time to repair itself after workouts. The more intense the workout, the longer it will take your body to recover. For example, if you're running several miles every other day, then you'll probably need at least two full days off each week to allow your muscles time to rebuild themselves before they can handle another challenging run session. A rest day is a perfect way to recharge your batteries, but it can be hard to tell if a person needs one. Here are some signs to look out for:

You're getting sick. Tiredness is often the first sign of illness. If you're feeling run down, it's probably best to take a break and let your body recover.

You can't remember what it feels like to be pain-free. If you're always in pain, this may mean that your body needs a break from whatever activity you're doing. This could mean taking more frequent breaks and stretching during long periods of sitting.

Struggling with concentration or memory problems. Focus and memory are linked with sleep quality; if someone is struggling with either of these things, they may need more sleep than usual or they may need a rest day so they can get better quality sleep at night (if they're getting enough sleep).

You wake up feeling sore every morning. If waking up with sore muscles is common for you, then this may be an indication that you need to take more rest days or reduce your physical activity levels. Soreness can also be caused by muscle imbalances — when one muscle group is stronger than another — if this might be an issue for you, get it corrected by working with a physical therapist who can prescribe exercises to help correct imbalances in muscle groups and improve joint mobility for greater comfort during movement.

You are constantly hungry (or thirsty). Hunger and thirst are both signs that your body needs food and water to function properly. If you find yourself constantly hungry, it could mean that you are over exercising and need to rest for your body to regain back energy.

Diet

Seniors can have trouble absorbing nutrients because their bodies are less able to use them. They are more prone to have medical conditions that affect their nutrition in comparison with the general population. Some reasons seniors have trouble maintaining a proper diet are:

Changes in taste and smell. Your sense of taste and smell may decline with age, which can reduce your enjoyment of foods. This can make it harder for you to notice when food is past its prime or spoiled.

Changes in digestion. As we get older, our bodies don't work as well at digesting certain nutrients and vitamins from food. This means that older adults need fewer calories than younger adults do in order to maintain their weight and avoid gaining weight as they age.

Changes in appetite. Older people often have smaller appetites than younger people do, even if they're not sick or frail. They also tend to eat less at meals than younger people do because they're less likely to be hungry between meals or late at night when they sleep.

Changes in the body's ability to absorb nutrients from food. The body's ability to absorb nutrients from food depends on several factors, such as how much vitamin B12 is stored in the liver and how much iron is stored in the blood.

Getting the right amount of nutrients is crucial for good health. But it can be difficult to get all the nutrients you need from food alone. If you're older or have certain health conditions, it's even more important to make sure you're getting enough vitamins and minerals each day.

The best way to make sure you're getting enough vitamins and minerals is by eating a variety of foods so that you get all the nutrients you need. A healthy diet includes plenty of fruits and vegetables, whole grains (such as brown rice), and legumes (such as beans). It also includes lean meats like fish or poultry; low-fat dairy products such as cheese or yogurt; and nuts and seeds in moderation because they are high in fat.

Older adults should also limit their intake of saturated fats (found mostly in animal products such as red meats) because these fats tend to increase blood cholesterol levels over time. In fact, a healthy diet is one of the best things you can do to maintain your health as you get older. The following sections discuss some key nutrients that are especially important for seniors and how to get enough of them in your diet. If you follow these steps, you can help keep yourself healthy:

Don't eat empty calories. Foods with empty calories are low in nutrients— such as chips, candy, and baked goods. They don't provide much nutrition for their calories so they're often called "junk food." If you do eat junk food occasionally, make sure it's not the main part of your meal or snack.

Take calcium and Vitamin D. Calcium is necessary for strong bones and teeth. It helps keep your bones strong so they don't break easily. It also helps prevent tooth decay by promoting remineralization (the process of rebuilding minerals on the surface of teeth).

Vitamin D helps with calcium absorption and bone health by increasing calcium stores in the body's soft tissues (including muscle) rather than just in the bones themselves. Vitamin D deficiency has been linked to osteoporosis and other bone diseases such as osteomalacia in older adults. The best way to get enough calcium is through food — not supplements — because foods provide other nutrients that work together with calcium.

Choose lean proteins, such as skinless chicken breast, or fish such as salmon or tuna, instead of red meat. Lean proteins provide many vitamins and minerals that contribute to good health in older adults. If you have trouble getting enough protein, you can use protein supplements such as powder shakes made with soy milk or other non-dairy milk. Or try adding a few nuts or seeds to your diet.

Choose whole grains over refined grains. Whole grains are high in fiber, which helps keep you full throughout the day, and they can help lower cholesterol levels and blood sugar levels—both risk factors for heart disease. They also have more vitamins and minerals than refined grains do, such as iron and magnesium (which helps control blood pressure). The best sources of whole grains include: 100 percent whole wheat bread or pasta; brown rice; quinoa; oatmeal; popcorn; and whole grain cereal (check nutrition labels to be sure it's 100 percent whole grain).

Eat plenty of fruits and vegetables. They're rich in vitamins A, C, and E; folate; potassium; iron; calcium; magnesium; carotenoids (plant pigments); flavonoids (antioxidants); lutein/zeaxanthin (which protect against eye diseases); lycopene (which protects against prostate cancer); selenium; omega-3 fatty acids (which protect brain function); zinc; chromium (which helps regulate blood sugar); copper; manganese and molybdenum (which help synthesize amino acids).

Drink plenty of water daily. About eight glasses for women and 10 for men — to keep your body hydrated throughout the day. Water is important because it carries nutrients to your cells and gets rid of waste products from your body. It also helps control blood pressure and body temperature.

Cut back on saturated fats (such as butter) by using olive oil instead on salads or in cooking when possible. Saturated fats raise cholesterol levels in your blood which increases your risk of heart disease.

Reduce sodium intake. Sodium is linked to high blood pressure, which increases your risk of heart disease, stroke, and kidney disease. To lower your sodium intake at home, look for low-sodium varieties of canned soups, low-sodium broths,and low-sugar ketchup at the grocery store or supermarket.

Choose low-fat or nonfat dairy products. Low-fat or nonfat dairy products are good sources of calcium and vitamin D, which are important for keeping bones strong as you age. Choose skim milk rather than 2% or whole milk when possible; it contains slightly less fat but still provides most of the nutrients found in whole milk — including calcium. You can also try soy milk or almond milk as an alternative to regular milk if you're trying to limit your intake of animal proteins like meat or eggs (which can be high in saturated fats).

Eat smaller portions. One of the biggest challenges for older adults is eating too much food at once. It's important to slow down and take time to chew your food well. This helps prevent choking and allows your body time to digest it properly. It's also a good idea to avoid eating right before bed because this can cause heartburn or indigestion if you sleep with a full stomach. Your body needs at least three hours after eating before bedtime so it has time to process all the food before sleep.

Keep a food diary to help you identify foods that trigger cravings. You might find that certain foods make you feel sick after eating them, or that they don't fill you up as much as others. If so, try to avoid those foods in your diet.

If necessary, ask your doctor about medication that may help calm or increase your appetite by boosting serotonin levels in the brain. Other medications can also be helpful for some people, such as those with diabetes or high blood pressure.

Training experience is always a debate surrounding exercise. The more you do it the better you get at it and make it look easy to an untrained eye. So more advanced movements should be easier than what we first attempt, right? That's true in some situations. But how much easier do we really want our exercises to be?

1. When Should You Modify Exercises?

If you have any pain or injuries in your joints or muscles, it's best to modify exercises that put pressure on these areas. For example, if you have knee pain, avoid lunges and squatting movements; if you have shoulder pain, avoid pushing movements; if you have wrist pain, avoid bicep curls and push-ups; etc.

2. What Should You Modify?

If there are certain parts of an exercise that are uncomfortable for you to perform — especially when compared to other people you are working out with— then it's time to modify it! For example: If you can only do 10 second planks but everyone else is doing 30 (or more!), then it might be time to modify it by putting your knees down.

3. Is the Exercise Safe?

Some exercises may be unsafe for certain people. For example, if you have knee pain, then you shouldn't perform squats because they put a lot of stress on your knees. To start slow and grow with time, you are free to follow this 12-week workout routine (note that the instructions for how to perform the exercises and the number of reps were covered earlier in the book).

Stretching

Stretching is often used as a warm-up for physical activities, such as running and resistance training, or as an injury prevention measure.

It can also be used to improve the flexibility of muscles, tendons, and joints in order to reduce the potential damage that may be caused by the shortening of these tissues during a workout. Stretches are performed before or after exercise, or at any other time when muscles are cold and tight.

And it is not just for people who want flexible joints; it can help with overall health. Many people who suffer from stiff muscles and joints are able to enjoy pain relief through regular stretching exercises.

A recent study found that stretching before exercise can decrease the risk of injuries among runners by up to 50 percent. Many people think that stretching is simply yoga. But there's a lot more to it than that.

Yoga and stretching are related, but they're not the same thing. Yoga is a system of exercise and meditation. It has its roots in religion, but people don't need to be religious to do it.

Stretching on the other hand, is a way of improving flexibility by holding poses for longer periods of time or by adding resistance (such as weights or bands) to your body parts.

Yoga focuses on developing strength and flexibility through postures (called asanas) and breathing techniques (called pranayama). The goal of yoga isn't just to improve flexibility; it's also about calming your mind and improving balance, endurance, and mental focus — all things that will help you perform better in sports and other activities where you need strong muscles along with good coordination and mental focus.

Unlike yoga, stretching is a crucial part of any workout routine. It not only helps you to avoid injury and improves your range of motion, but it also helps the body warm up for exercise. Warming up increases blood flow to the muscles, which means that there's more oxygen and nutrients available for your muscles to use during exercise.

It also helps to loosen the muscles, which improves their elasticity and reduces the risk of injury. The best way to stretch is to hold each position for 10 to 15 seconds before repeating on the other side. You should feel a slight pull in your muscles without experiencing pain. Don't bounce or strain against the stretch — just allow gravity to do its job! Here are some of the most common stretches you can do before a workout:

Quadriceps stretch

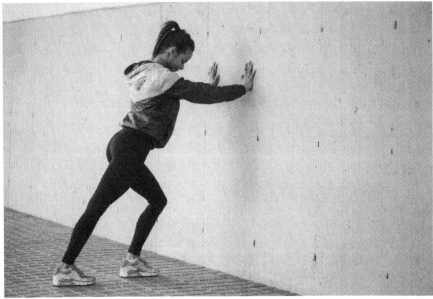

Stand facing a wall with both feet flat on the floor and about an inch away from it. Lower your upper body toward the wall until you feel a stretch in your front thigh muscle (the quadriceps). Hold for 20 seconds, then relax. Repeat three times on each leg.

Hamstring stretch

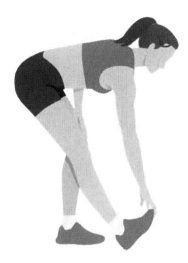

Stand with one foot forward and one foot back (or sit on a chair), keeping both knees slightly bent so that your lower back doesn't arch too much in either direction (a sign of poor form). Slowly bend from your hips toward the floor until you feel the tension in your hamstrings. Hold for 20 seconds, then relax.

Sitting extension stretch

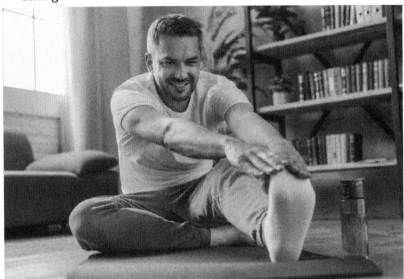

Sit on the floor with one leg extended straight out in front of you and the other bent with your foot flat on the floor. Pull your toes toward you, then push them away from you until you feel a stretch in the front of your thigh. Hold for 30 seconds, then switch legs and repeat.

Calf stretch

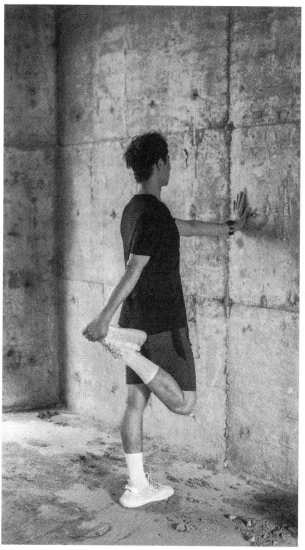

Stand facing a wall with both feet approximately 12 inches away from it and parallel to each other. Rest one hand on the wall while bending one leg behind you so that your heel is touching the wall. Lean forward until you feel a gentle stretch in your calves. Hold for 10 seconds, then switch legs and repeat 3 times per leg.

Stretching after a workout is especially important because it helps to relax the body and muscles. After exercise, your body releases endorphins, which are natural painkillers that make you feel good.

When you stretch after a workout, these endorphins remain in the bloodstream longer than if you had not stretched at all.

Stretching helps to increase blood flow to all parts of the body. This improves circulation and helps remove lactic acid from your muscles, which reduces soreness after exercise. A warm muscle has more blood vessels open, allowing more blood to flow through it. This means that more oxygen is delivered to working muscles and nutrients are delivered to damaged muscle fibers.

As you stretch, your body releases chemicals called endorphins — also known as painkillers — and other hormones that relieve stress and reduce anxiety. Stretching can also help you relax after a stressful day or bring about sleepiness if done before bedtime.

But be aware that it can cause injury if you do too much too quickly or if you have an underlying medical condition such as arthritis or fibromyalgia (a disorder characterized by widespread musculoskeletal pain and tenderness). If you're not sure how much stretching is right for you, talk with your doctor first. The most common post workout stretching positions are the cobra stretch and the child pose as they prove to be more effective on your upper body. You can also, however, practice these three other stretches for the lower body after your workout:

Butterfly

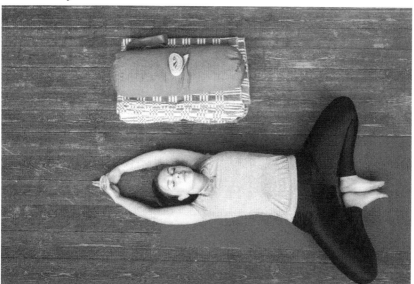

To perform the butterfly, lie on your back with your knees bent and feet flat on the floor. Bring your hands over your head. Bend both feet and move them as close as possible to your groin area until you feel a stretch in your inner thighs; hold for 30 seconds then let go.

Standing Quadricep Stretch

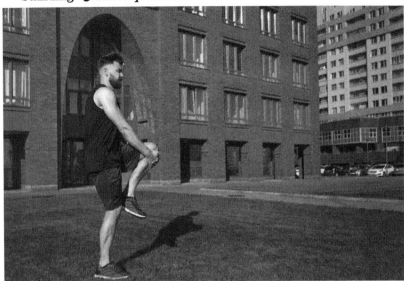

Begin this quadriceps (in the front of the thigh) by standing with legs slightly open. Bend your right leg and hold on to the foot in front of your chest, keeping weight on the heel. Straighten the leg in front of you and keep the back straight. Hold for 20 to 30 seconds, then repeat on the other side.

Seated Spinal Twist

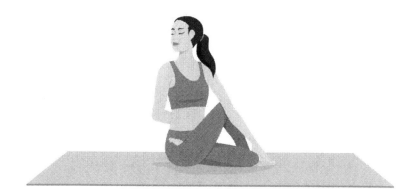

This is another great pose for beginners. You can do this pose seated on the floor or in a chair if you're more comfortable with your back supported. Sit up tall with your legs crossed in front of you and your feet about hip-width apart. Place your right hand behind your right leg and turn towards it until you feel a stretch through your left side. Take this time to breathe deeply into the stretch. Repeat on the other side.

12-week beginners resistance band workout

NOTE: For the best results always exhale while doing the workout and inhale when going back to the starting position.

Exercise Time: 15 - 20 minutes per session

Exercise volume: 4 days a week

Woodchopper

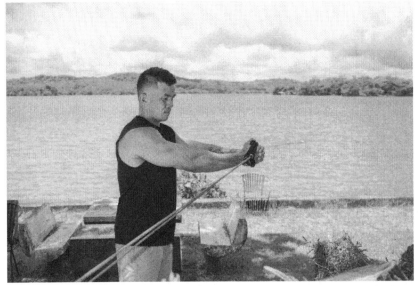

To do this exercise, hold both ends of the resistance band with the corresponding hand and stand with feet shoulder-width apart and knees slightly bent. Bring one end of the band up to chest level while twisting at the hips to bring in the opposite side (the other end) behind you. You should feel tension on your obliques as you twist. Then bring it back down to chest level and repeat for 2 reps before switching sides.

Triceps kickbacks

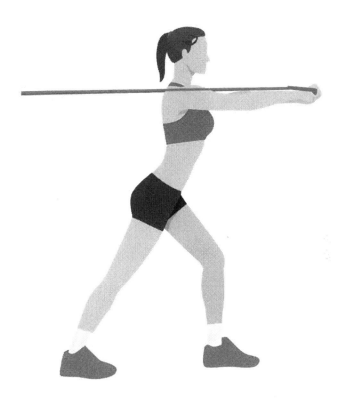

Stand facing away from the anchor point of the resistance band, holding it with both hands in front of your body at chest level. Your palms should be facing inward towards each other. Bend both elbows 90 degrees so that they are at right angles with your upper arms, then slowly straighten them back out again until they're fully extended but not locked out (this will be about 45 degrees). When performing this exercise, make sure that you don't allow your elbows to come together behind your body as this will cause unnecessary stress on them and could lead to injury.

Pull-apart exercise

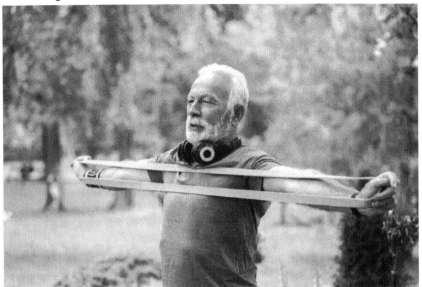

This is a great exercise for developing shoulders and arms. To do it, stand up and keep your legs slightly apart and knees slightly bent. Hold one end of the band in the corresponding hand so that it's taut and there's no slack in the middle. Bring your hands together so that they're touching at chest level with palms facing each other. Then slowly pull them apart until they are at ear level with palms facing away from you at all times.

Overhead pull-apart

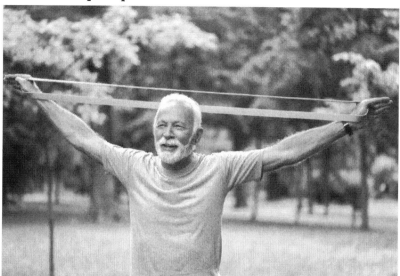

Stand facing with your feet together and knees slightly bent. Grab both ends of the band with one hand on each handle and raise them up overhead until both arms are extended straight above you. Slowly pull the handles apart while keeping your arms straight overhead. Once they're fully stretched out overhead, slowly return them to their original position above your head. Repeat this 8-10 times for one set and perform 3-4 sets total.

Bicep curl

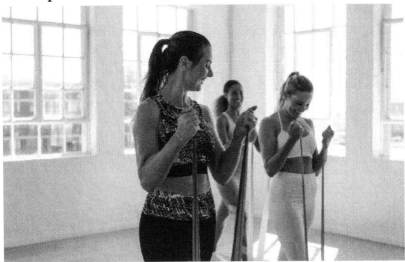

Stand with feet hip-width apart, knees slightly bent, and back straight. Hold the center of a resistance band in each hand, palms facing down with wrists bent back and elbows slightly bent. Arms should be extended out in front of you (you may have to adjust your grip on the band as you progress). Squeeze your shoulder blades together as you bring your hands toward your shoulders until they almost touch behind you. Slowly return to the starting position.

Bent-over row

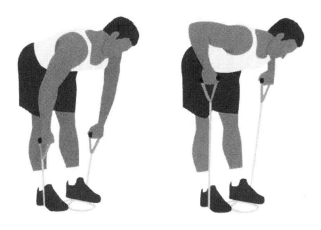

To perform this exercise, stand straight with your legs slightly open and hold the band in both hands with your arms extended at chest height. Your palms should be facing down and your elbows should be bent at 90 degrees. Slowly pull the band towards your chest by bending at the waist until you feel a stretch in your shoulders, then slowly return to starting position. Repeat for eight to 12 repetitions.

Standing side taps

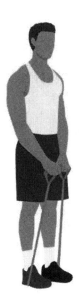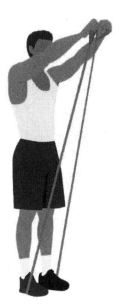

Start by standing with your feet together, holding the band in both hands. Squeeze your shoulder blades together and hold the band with your arms straight out in front of you at chest level. Pull the band over your head, keeping your legs straight and knees locked. Return to the starting position and repeat 10 times.

Overhead press

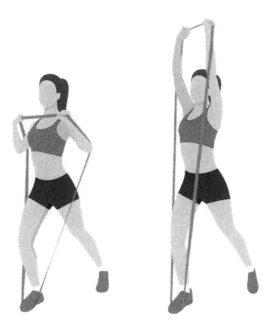

Start with one foot forward, standing on top of the band, and the other foot back behind you. Switch your grip, grabbing the handles from underneath so that your palms are facing forward and away from you. Start by holding the handles at shoulder height. Then add pressure over your head, extending both arms straight above you. Repeat 8-10 times.

Standing lateral band walk

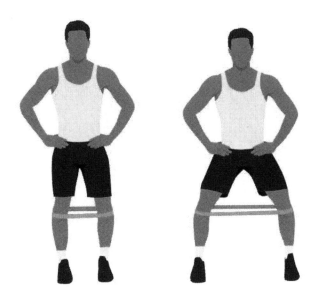

Place feet in a resistance band with both feet slightly open. Grab the hips and slightly bend your body so that you feel the tension in the band. Keep your back straight and shoulders down as you rotate your hips outward. Now open one leg outward and then step inward with that same leg until both feet are together again. That's one rep! Repeat for 8 reps per side before switching legs and repeating again for an additional 8 reps per side.

Standing banded squat

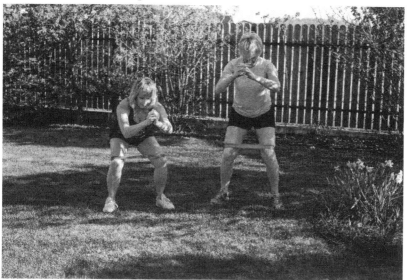

This is a great exercise to start with, as it's simple and easy to do. Simply wrap the band around your knees You can then squat down and stand up again while keeping the tension in the band. You can also do this exercise while holding on to a chair if you have balance issues, just make sure to keep your knee soft! This exercise will help improve your core stability, which makes it a great addition to any workout routine.

Banded bridge

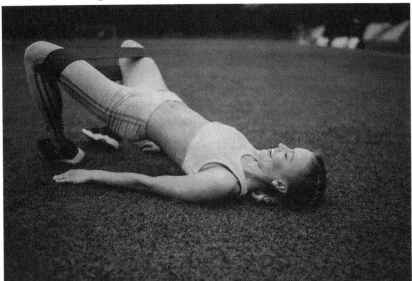

To do this exercise, place a resistance band around your hips and lie on your back with your knees bent and feet flat on the floor. Then squeeze your glutes and drive through your heels as you press up into a bridge position. Hold for one count at the top of the movement before lowering back down to starting position. If you're using an extra-thick band, you'll need to make sure it's anchored securely so it doesn't slip or slide off during your set. If you're using a lighter band, try using two hands to anchor the band so it doesn't slip or slide off during your set.

Intermediate: Week 4 - 12+

In weeks 9 -12+, you will do a split workout.

NOTE: For the best results always exhale while doing the workout and inhale when going back to the starting position.

Exercise Time: 15 - 20 minutes per session

Exercise volume: 5 days a week

NOTE: Do 3 full body workouts and 2 split workout sessions a week.

Arm & Leg Day
Overhead Pull-Apart

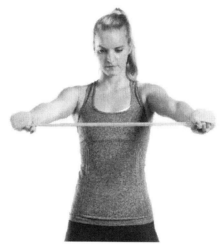

The overhead pull-apart is similar to the push-up, but you're using resistance bands instead of body weight to challenge your body even further. To perform this exercise, hold the band with both hands above your head and pull.

Front Raise

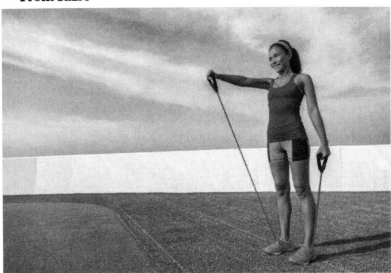

Stand with your feet shoulder-width apart and hold the ends of the resistance band. With your arms bent at 90 degrees and palms facing forward, raise your one arm out in front of you until it is parallel to the floor. Your elbows should be flexed at 90° and your forearms should be vertical throughout the exercise. Slowly return to the starting position and repeat for desired reps on both arms.

Pull-Apart

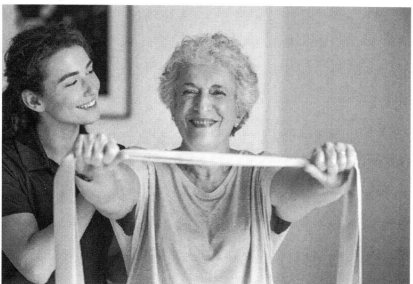

This is a great exercise to work your back and shoulders. The key to this exercise is to not just go through the motions but really focus on squeezing those muscles. It's also important to keep your back straight and your shoulders down and away from your ears.

Bent-Over T Flies

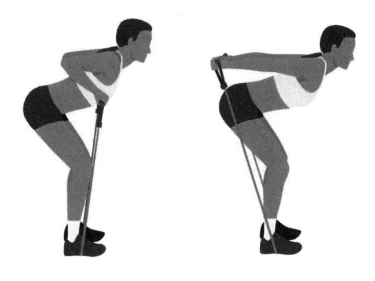

To perform this exercise, start by holding the handles of the resistance band. Bend over at the hips and keep your back straight. Your arms should be bent down from your shoulders with palms facing forward. Now raise your arms back until they are almost parallel to the floor. You should feel this in your chest and upper back. Lower your arms back down to starting position and repeat for reps or time.

Leg Lifts

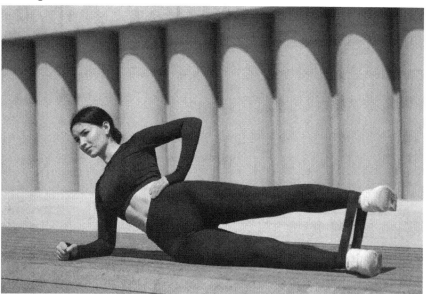

Put a resistance band around both ankles while lying sideways on the floor. Lift your right leg up as high as possible without straining. Hold for two seconds then slowly lower your leg down to the starting position. Repeat this movement with your other leg. Perform three sets of 15 reps on each side.

Squats

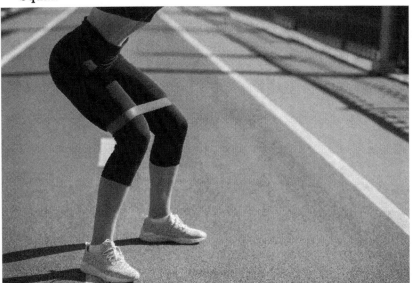

The squat is one of the best exercises for building strength and muscle mass. It works your entire lower body, and it's particularly effective for targeting your glutes, quads, and hamstrings. By adding a resistance band to this exercise, you can increase the intensity of the movement while also improving your balance and stability. Do 8-10 reps for 2 sets.

Lateral Band Walk

LATERAL STEPS & SQUATS
WITH RESISTANCE BAND

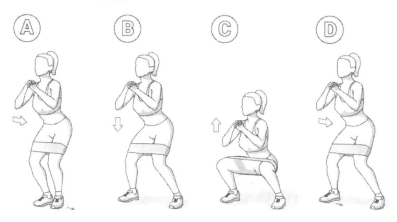

This is an effective way to work on lateral stability, which is important for good posture and preventing injury. Stand with your feet together and the band wrapped around your thighs. Step out to the right with your other leg,and follow with the other. Slowly move sideways while slightly squatting until you feel a moderate stretch on the outside of your right thigh. Hold for two seconds for each full step you take, then step back to the center with both feet. Repeat this movement 10 times.

Glute Kickbacks

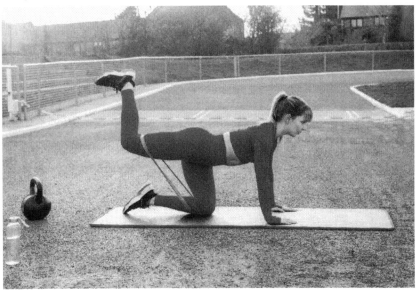

The gluteus maximus is a large muscle that makes up the buttocks. This exercise targets the glutes while building strength in the hamstrings and lower back.

With all fours on a mat, place a resistance band placed at knee level. Keep your arms straight and one leg on the floor while raising the other leg. The resistance band should be pulled tight, so you feel the tension in your glutes when you kick back.

Keeping your chest lifted and core engaged, kick back one leg at a time as far as you can, then return to starting position by extending your leg behind you without locking out your knee. Focus on keeping your hips square and not arching or leaning forward. Perform 10 reps on each side before moving on to the next exercise.

Shoulders & Back Day

Side raises

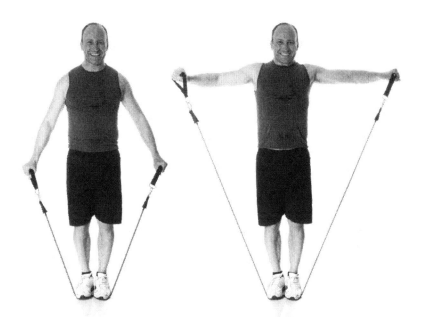

Hold resistance bands with both hands, palms facing your body. Raise your arms outwards until they are parallel to the floor, keeping them at shoulder height. Slowly lower your arms back down to starting position. Repeat 15 times on both sides.

Upright row

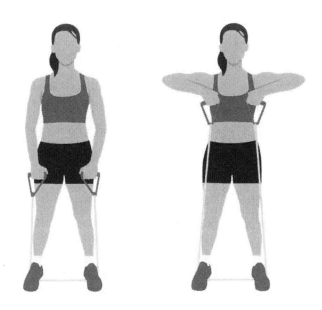

Grasp the handles of the band, holding them with both hands at waist level and slightly wider than shoulder-width apart. Position your arms straight out with elbows bent 90 degrees. Your palms should be facing each other. Now raise both arms up towards the ceiling until they are almost pointing to the ground while keeping your elbows slightly bent. Return to starting position and repeat for 10 to 12 repetitions with both arms.

Bent-over rows

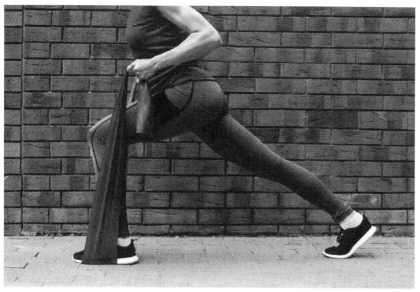

To perform bent-over rows with a resistance band, stand with your feet apart and hold one end of the band with the corresponding hand at arm's length in front of your body. Keep your elbows close to your sides as you bend forward at the waist until it feels like you're about to lose balance. Place one foot forward and the other foot behind you.

Step on the band with the foot that you placed forward, then pull the band up toward your chest while keeping elbows close to the sides (you should feel this in your back muscles). Reverse movement back down until arms are straight out again.

Straight-arm pulldown

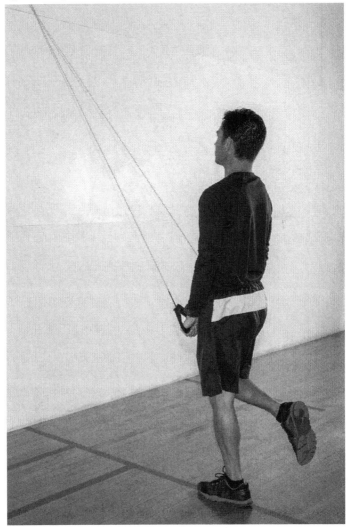

Attach the long tube band to a door or anchor on the wall, making sure it is secure. While standing up, maintain the same distance between your arms and torso throughout the movement. Slowly pull the handles of the band down toward your side until it touches your hip before returning to the start position. Repeat with the opposite arm to complete one rep.

Full Body 2x

One-arm biceps curl

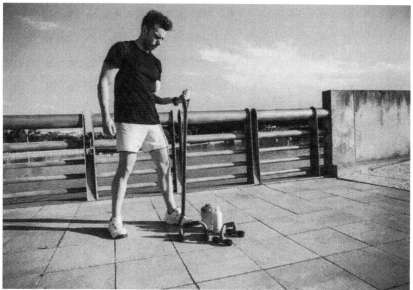

Stand with your legs slightly apart, knees slightly bent, hold the resistance band with your right hand and step on the other side of the band with your right leg. This is your starting position. Then raise your right arm up in front of you until it's parallel to the floor. Slowly return to the starting position and repeat on the other side.

Side-lying hip abduction

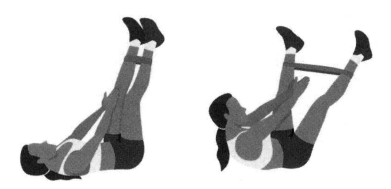

Lie on your side with your legs in the air out in front of you, knees slightly bent, and feet together. Wrap the band around both legs just above your ankles, then pull your legs apart as much as your body allows you to. Keep your core engaged, and abs are drawn in as you keep your legs lifted. You should feel this in your outer thighs. Repeat on both sides until you've completed 5-8 reps per side.

Wall squat

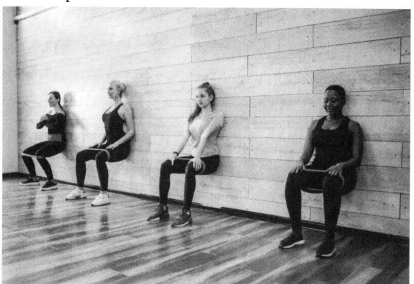

Attach the resistance band around your ankles, knees, or thighs. The higher up you attach it, the more difficult the exercise will be. Rest your back against a wall and take a squat position. Keep your core tight and chest up as you hinge at the hips and bend forward at the waist until your buttocks are parallel to the floor. Hold this position for 5 counts before returning to standing. Repeat 2 times.

Splitter

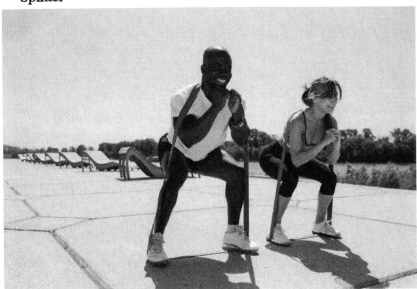

To do this exercise, you will need a long band. The wider the band, the easier it is to do this exercise. Set up in a split stance with your feet apart at least as wide as your shoulders. Step on the band and secure the other end above your shoulders. Your elbows should be bent slightly and pointing out to the side with palms facing forward or up toward the ceiling at about shoulder height.

Step forward into a squat position, keeping knees bent 90 degrees or less with both feet on the floor. Return to starting position by straightening the elbows back out in front of the body while stepping back into starting position. Repeat this motion until you have completed 5 reps per side.

Glute bridge

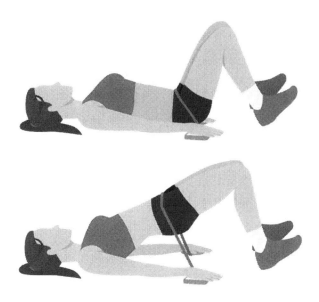

Start lying on your back with your feet flat on the floor and your knees bent at 90 degrees, holding onto each end of the resistance band with both hands. Your arms should be extended while holding the band across your pelvic area (depending on how much weight you want to use). Press through your heels into the floor as you squeeze your glutes together to lift your hips off the ground until they form a straight line from knees to shoulders. Pause for 2 seconds at the top of the movement before lowering back down slowly until your butt touches the ground again.

Squat to overhead press

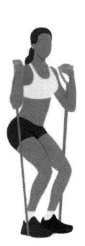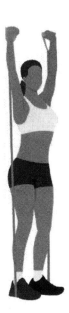

Go down into a squat, keeping our head up. And then come back up and press over your head with the band. As you come back down, push out at the bottom of the squat so that you get some good extension at the top of your range of motion. Make sure to keep your hips straight down and not moving side-to-side as well. So keep your heels flat on the ground and push out at the bottom of the squat for a great posterior chain exercise using resistance bands!

Lateral walk/steps

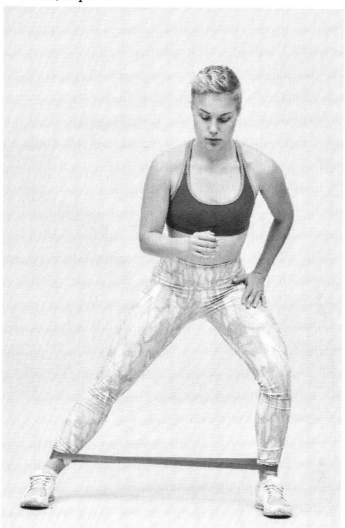

This exercise helps strengthen the muscles on both sides of your body. It also helps in improving balance while walking, running, or jogging. To do this exercise, stand straight with feet hip-width apart, and bend one knee while keeping the other foot flat on the ground. Walk sideways with one foot at a time while keeping the knee raised up all throughout the motion. Do 10-12 repetitions with each leg before switching sides.

Strive for success

The more you live your life, the more you realize that there are so many opportunities to do something different and make a change. The first thing you need to do is develop a positive attitude.

This is the foundation of all confidence-building activities. Being aware of your emotions and thoughts is important because they can affect your actions. For example, if you are feeling sad or depressed, it will be hard for you to get up and start doing your daily workout session.

So, to build self-confidence, you need to start by changing your thoughts and feelings about yourself. When you think positively about yourself and your abilities, you will find it easier to take action towards achieving your goals.

Another thing that helps with gaining self-confidence is having a strong sense of fulfillment in life. Seniors who have this kind of fulfillment tend to be happier and more resilient when faced with challenges or setbacks because they are driven by something greater than themselves, such as family, religion, or community service work. There are many ways to gain the right confidence and accomplish your exercise goals. Here are a few suggestions:

1. Set goals for yourself that you want to achieve by keeping a daily journal. For example, if you want to gain muscle, list the steps that need to be taken to reach your goal, and then check them off as they are completed. This will help keep you focused on your goal

and also give you a sense of accomplishment when each step is completed. Write how you felt for the day and whether you exercised or not. Journaling significantly increases your chances of success.

2. If you have ever done something difficult or challenging but ultimately rewarding (e.g., finally completing 30-second plank), think back on that experience and remember how proud you felt once you had accomplished it. Try to recapture those feelings by thinking about what it was like when you first started learning to do something new and difficult. However, you knew deep down inside that you would eventually succeed because you always do what's best for yourself!

3. Start doing things on your own without relying on others so much for help, advice, or reassurance (e.g., asking a friend what they think before starting your exercise journey). Once we practice doing this enough, we'll become more confident in our abilities without the need for constant validation. This tip doesn't count for your doctor or healthcare provider, as you should always ask them for help or advice when needed.

The first step to succeeding in this new journey is overcoming mental barriers. The key is to focus on the end result. Do your best to ignore what other people think about seniors gaining muscle by pulling some bands around. Instead, focus on becoming the best and healthiest version of yourself.

The benefits of exercising with resistance bands are numerous, but most importantly, it can help you live a longer and healthier life. Working out improves cardiovascular health, reduces stress, and promotes better sleep habits. When it comes to exercise, age is just a number.

"The biggest challenge is mental," says Dr. Andrew Hunt, a sports medicine physician who coaches cross-country runners (Brigham and Women's Hospital in Boston). "You have to overcome everything telling you not to do it."

Hunt says he sees this every year with his runners – many of whom are beginners when they start training for cross-country in September. They go through several phases before learning how to run properly – starting with walking and then building up their endurance over weeks or months until they can run for longer periods without stopping for rest breaks or pain relief medication like ibuprofen or acetaminophen.

Eating healthy and exercising more often is often much easier said than done. Many people have had bad experiences with diets and workouts because it all starts with the mind. Getting up from the couch and going for a workout can feel more daunting than it should. It takes more than just motivation to get yourself in good shape; it also requires mental strength and discipline.

The best way to overcome these mental barriers is to start by focusing on what you need to do daily. Take it one day at a time. *Don't get discouraged.*

Here's another book by Scott Hamrick
that you might like

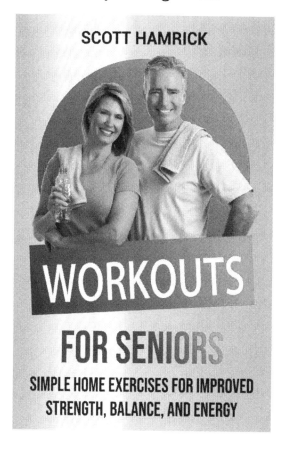

Free Bonuses from Scott Hamrick

Hi seniors!

My name is Scott Hamrick, and first off, I want to THANK YOU for reading my book.

Now you have a chance to join my exclusive "workout for seniors" email list so you can get the ebook below for free as well as the potential to get more ebooks for seniors for free! Simply click the link below to join.

P.S. Remember that it's 100% free to join the list.

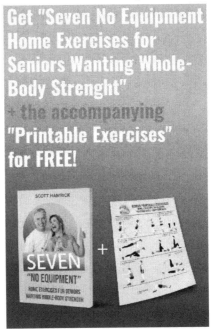

Access your free bonuses here:

https://livetolearn.lpages.co/resistance-band-workout-for-seniors-paperback/

Printed in Great Britain
by Amazon

18330205R00097